THE
PERFECT
ORGASM

Also by Joan Elizabeth Lloyd

Nonfiction
Nice Couples Do
If It Feels Good
Come Play With Me
Now and Forever, Let's Make Love
52 Saturday Nights
Totally Private
Naughty Secrets

Fiction
Black Satin
The Pleasures of Jessica Lynn
The Love Flower
Velvet Whispers
Slow Dancing
Midnight Butterfly
The Price of Pleasure
Never Enough
Club Fantasy
Night After Night
Bedtime Stories for Lovers
Naughty Bedtime Stories

THE
PERFECT
ORGASM

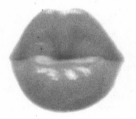

How to Get It, How to Give It

JOAN ELIZABETH LLOYD

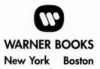

WARNER BOOKS
New York Boston

This book is intended for use by adults who are informed and want to invigorate and maintain a great sexual relationship. The author is not medically trained, and the reader is reminded that following these guidelines and new ideas is voluntary and at the reader's own discretion. The positions and methodology presented herein are safe and satisfying for most adult men and women, however, every individual is different and you should not undertake any position or technique that is not suitable to your physical condition. You should consult a health care professional with any questions. Certain acts described in this book are illegal in some states and you should be aware of the laws in your area.

Copyright © 2005 by Joan Elizabeth Lloyd
All rights reserved.

Warner Books

Time Warner Book Group
1271 Avenue of the Americas, New York, NY 10020
Visit our Web site at www.twbookmark.com.

Printed in the United States of America

First Edition: July 2005
10   9   8   7   6   5   4   3   2   1

Library of Congress Cataloging-in-Publication Data
Lloyd, Joan Elizabeth.
    The perfect orgasm: how to get it, how to give it/Joan Elizabeth Lloyd.
        p. cm.
    ISBN 0-446-69267-0
    1. Sexual excitement. 2. Orgasm. 3. Sex instruction. I. Title.
    HQ31.L664 2005
    613.9'6 –dc22   2004030273

CONTENTS

INTRODUCTION

PERFECT ORGASMS

DURING MY FIFTEEN YEARS OF WRITING BOOKS
about sexuality, running a very active Web site with forums for visitors
to express their views, and answering questions about lovemaking,
I've thought a lot about orgasms. I've finally distilled my thoughts
into this riddle:

Why is an orgasm like a sandwich?

Silly, I admit, but a sandwich is actually an apt analogy. To see
why, let's answer the riddle:

First, a sandwich is built of lots of separate parts, some more
important than others. You need a foundation, the bread, be it
Wonder white, caraway-seeded rye, pita, or a flat bread for a
wrap. This is probably the most underappreciated part, the basis
of a great sandwich. It's also the most important because it's the
only way to get it to your mouth.

Sandwiches vary in complexity from the old favorite, peanut
butter on white, through ham and cheese with mustard and lettuce, to the Italian combo with four kinds of meat, two cheeses,
lettuce, tomatoes, hot peppers, and olives, topped with oil and
vinegar.

The same sandwich doesn't satisfy the same way every day.
Today you might be in the mood for roast beef on a roll; tomorrow it's Muenster cheese, salami, black olives, and mustard. The
following day cream cheese and jelly or an old-fashioned cheese-
burger suits best.

Sometimes a sandwich needs a side dish, whether it be well-done french fries or coleslaw and a pickle. The next day you may just want a quick veggie wrap.

Orgasms are the same in many ways. Lots of pieces go into building a satisfying climax, and the building blocks vary from encounter to encounter. What was fabulous yesterday—long, slow lovemaking in the bedroom with the lights out—might not be the most exciting today—a hot quickie on the dining room table—or tomorrow, when mutual masturbation or a blindfold might be just the thing.

What constitutes the perfect orgasm? I asked visitors to my Web site to describe their concept of a perfect orgasm. As I expected, the answers varied widely.

A forty-two-year-old man wrote:

The Perfect Orgasm for me is a very *hungry* orgasm.

Since my wife and I have sex (intercourse or mutual masturbation) on a fairly regular basis, if we don't get any for about a week (due to illness or our busy schedules) we tend to get really horny. Both body and mind yearn for the sensual buildup, the plateau, and the orgasmic release.

Speaking for myself, if I haven't had a ripping orgasm in many days I start getting more spontaneous erections. I feel the need for a warm, wet mouth, a hot, pulsing pussy, or my own loving touch. When I finally get the opportunity for satisfaction, instead of just rushing through it to scratch the incredible itch, I try to draw out the pleasures and savor each and every sensation. Whether it's my wife's mouth, her hungry vagina, or my fist, when my cock is finally getting some attention, I'm in another world. I concentrate on how good each movement feels and I float toward the edge of orgasm, and I can linger there as long as possible before taking my final, ultimate pleasure.

The perfect orgasm makes my whole body shake. When I feel the release from deep inside me, an electric glow runs from one end of me to the other. Perfect orgasms are mind-blowing, totally satisfying, and they really wear you out!

A thirty-seven-year-old man wrote:

I believe the prefect orgasm can only be achieved when both people are true lovers. You need that perfect formula to experience the ultimate mind-blowing orgasm. You need to use all your senses: the feel of soft touches, the aroma of sweet smells, the intoxicating sight of her beauty, hearing her moans, all add to the sense of deep love I have for my wife. Then I add just a touch of fantasy or sexy thoughts of her erotic body.

A perfect orgasm starts from the first look of want, desire, and lust, progresses to wet sloppy kisses and touching of her soft, warm, smooth feminine skin. Whispering "I love you" softly in her ear, allowing my breath to do some magic flows from there. The more slowly I go, the faster the world around me disappears.

Curious about her answer, I asked my wife the question and she said, "If an orgasm is really perfect I will experience long multiple climaxes, ending with complete satisfaction and euphoria. The period close to actual orgasm can last for almost an hour. That sensation of being in the moment, with total concentration on sensual pleasure before orgasm, can heighten the actual climax, making all of my nerve endings feel everything more intensely. I become a purely sexual being."

A *twenty-eight-year-old woman* wrote:

Perfect orgasm? I know you want me to tell you about one, but I've had so many it's difficult to choose. I love to have sex and I've had great sex with several men in lots of different places and ways. If I had to make a choice, I guess I'd say it was being tied up, unable to take part, just being serviced by my boyfriend at the time. Is that very selfish?

A *thirty-five-year-old man* wrote:

A couple of years ago my wife and I went to a convention with several other co-workers. When we checked in we discovered, to our delight, that we had been upgraded to a suite at no extra charge. We went up to the room and, since we'd been traveling for half a day, I got undressed and hopped into the shower for a few minutes. As I stood under the hot water, it dawned on me that I was really wasting a golden opportunity, so I called my wife who quickly agreed with my assessment. It took only a moment for her to strip off her clothes and join me in our "shower built for two." I grabbed her in an embrace, deep-kissing her while pushing her up against the tile wall under the cascade of steamy water.

My cock slowly started to harden against her pussy as I massaged her breasts and moved my mouth down to suck her tits and flick her erect nipples with my tongue. She had already reached down and begun playing with my dangling balls and lightly tweaking my swollen dickhead. When I couldn't hold back any longer I had to turn her around and fucked her hot, wet pussy from the rear. The combination of pumping my cock in and out of her and the water cascading over us was making us both wild with ecstasy and since no one could hear us we were both yelling with abandon. I could tell she was coming so I just let loose. I'll never forget that amazingly powerful orgasm, both mine and hers. Perfect? Yeah, but not the only perfect one I've ever had. Thank God!

A thirty-one-year-old man wrote:

For me to have a perfect orgasm, I have to be inactive, on the receiving end only. The best way—perhaps the only way—is for me to receive a blow job while lying completely relaxed, flat on my back. My orgasm needs time to build and I can't rush it. I must relax and feel the pressure start to build and let it come of its own accord. When it happens it feels as if my whole body is coming out the head of my penis. This of course doesn't happen very often, but when it does, it's heaven.

A thirty-three-year-old man wrote:

I can't say that I've ever experienced a "perfect" orgasm, but I have one great one that comes to mind. I had only been out with this particular young woman a few times and this was going to be the first time we'd spent the night together. She'd agreed to take a motorcycle ride with me to a friend's house in the country and stay over. Since she'd never been on a bike before I stopped at the Harley shop where I'd purchased my bike and picked up a leather jacket, chaps, boots, and a helmet for her. The day was perfect, bright sun and a cool breeze. She took to the bike as though she'd been riding for years and we had a wonderful day. I have to admit that, although I admired the scenery, I also kept thinking about the night to come.

We arrived at the lake just before sunset and sat for a few minutes just gazing at the colors as the sun dropped behind the distant mountains. Eventually she grabbed her tote bag and, after I dropped my jacket and some gear inside, I went back out to the bike for the saddlebags with my stuff.

When I returned, I was met by my passenger wearing nothing but the new leather gear I'd purchased for her. She pushed me back into a big smoking chair, undid the buttons on my jeans, and straddled my hips, lowering her exposed pussy onto my already hard-as-steel cock. I still remember the noise that my leather made against her chaps and to this day the smell of leather brings back that memory.

As she bobbed up and down the length of my erection, I eased back into the plush chair and grasped at her firm tits as they jutted out from her open leather jacket. To maintain her balance, she held on to the bandanna I was wearing around my neck with one hand while she worked her clit with the other. Every time I'd moan, or make any noise at all, she'd gasp, "Don't come yet, don't come yet." As she neared orgasm, she slowed her pace a bit, preferring more to stroke herself just over the head of my dick.

When I thought I'd climax from the excitement

of it, she started to come. I could feel the contractions of her pussy around the tip of my erection and I exploded inside of her. It felt like I was coming forever.

Like I said in the beginning, maybe not yet perfect, but oh, so memorable.

A thirty-seven-year-old man wrote:

Several years ago, on Good Friday, my wife and I went shopping on her lunch break to get her a new dress for Easter. We were holding hands as we walked through the mall, and even though at the time we'd been married for twelve years, we were acting sort of like teenagers with hormones raging. Why we were so hot I'll never know and, sadly, I've not been able to duplicate that feeling since.

We went into one store to look at dresses, and she found a few she liked so she took them into a dressing room. Since the store wasn't busy, and I was standing there thinking of her stripping down to her skivvies, I got the urge to join her. I looked around to make sure no one saw me, then slipped into the room she was in.

She was standing there in her bra and panties and without hesitation I started kissing her on the lips, and then on the special place at the side of her neck that I know drives her crazy. Before long she was kissing me back with as much heat as I felt. I peeled her panties off, sat her down on the bench in the room, and started kissing her where it counted. She muttered a few protests about being caught, but both of us were too far into it to quit. I could tell she was getting ready to come because she was holding my head hard against her and trying to stifle the noises she was making. She was jerking around that little bench, but kept my head tight against her for what seemed like forever.

When she finally let me up for air, I unbuckled my pants, and she helped me push them down to my ankles. She said she wanted me inside her. Now! When I entered her, she wrapped her legs around my back to hold on. Just a couple of thrusts and she came, followed quickly by my climax.

Eventually I got my clothes readjusted, and took my wonderful wife back to work. This was just the beginning of what was to become one of the most romantic weekends of our marriage and a most perfect orgasm.

A thirty-six-year-old man wrote:

It's hard for me to pick one orgasm that I can say is perfect—I'm still waiting for *absolutely* perfect—but there is one that I recall as very close.

It was about seven years ago, and I had a brief thing going with a quiet, nice girl, with a calmness about her and breasts that were, ah . . . let's just say not very calming.

Anyway, sex quickly progressed from kisses to heavy petting. One night we got to the point where she gave me oral sex. She made no big deal of it, just gave me pleasure. No big show or anything, just the thing itself. I don't really remember the details of what and how but out of her lengthy, calm, mellow sucking an amazing orgasm took me by surprise. I think I ejaculated a lot. It was a long, powerful climax with me bouncing and making a lot of noise. No thinking through all of it, no evaluating her skills—*Man, she's doing this and that really well* as we guys are prone to do—no strong emotions either. Just good sex. Just being there and receiving my pleasure.

A *twenty-three-year-old woman wrote:*

I hate to admit this but the most perfect orgasm I ever had was with a perfect stranger—a very perfect stranger.

Several months ago I was invited to a party thrown by some friends and, since I was between relationships, I decided to go because it might be fun to check out the single guys. As the evening progressed one guy stood out from the rest. He wasn't particularly good looking but he had "those eyes"—the sexy ones that look at you as if to say, *I know what you're wearing under those clothes and I want some.*

Well, by late in the evening I wanted some too. I was so hot I thought I'd spontaneously combust. I slipped upstairs to use a more private bathroom than the one on the main floor and maybe masturbate to calm my body. I closed the door and finished the business part of the visit, then stood up to wash my hands.

Suddenly the door behind me opened. I guess I'd forgotten to lock it but I thought I was alone on the upper floor. Anyway, who slipped in behind me but "sexy eyes." I didn't even know his name. I could see him in the mirror, his face a mask of desire. His look made me still hotter.

He pressed his front against my back and there was no doubt of his interest. The hard ridge banging against the small of my back left no doubt. He said nothing, just lifted my sweater and scooped my breasts from my bra. He rolled and pulled at my nipples until I thought I'd explode. Soon he had my skirt up, my panties down, and a condom on his raging hard-on.

Then he was inside me. I usually have great self-control but not that night. I stuffed my fist into my mouth to keep from screaming as he pounded into me. I thought I'd come forever but all too soon our bodies calmed. Still silent, he cleaned up and slipped back out the door. By the time I got back downstairs he was gone and I've not seen him since. I keep hoping I'll run into him again, but maybe that would be a letdown. For the moment, he forms the basis of many wonderful fantasies.

A fifty-year-old man wrote:

I went to Reno, Nevada, in the early 1970s with some friends and one evening they took me to a place called the Mustang Ranch. Although I was far from a virgin, this was the first time I've ever been to a place like that. I was both overwhelmed and euphoric and ended up choosing an escort who reminded me of a girl whom I had always had fantasies about in high school.

We went to her room, undressed, and she gave me wonderful oral stimulation. In my mind I just went away, only feeling, not thinking of anything. My excitement grew to such an extent that the next thing I remember is her straddling me and my having the most powerful, thrusting orgasm of my life. It centered in my cock and balls, without any thoughts of any kind. Afterward she grinned,

looked into my eyes, and said, "I think I got you."
Boy, she sure did.

A *twenty-eight-year-old woman wrote:*

My best and most perfect orgasm happened on
my honeymoon. My husband and I had lived
together for about a year before we got married
so the honeymoon was really a much-needed
vacation for both of us. We spent the entire week
just being together with no distractions. One
evening we went to the small nightclub in the
hotel. My husband ordered a bottle of champagne and we danced. We did some fast stuff but
we also did the kind of slow-dancing you see in
the movies. My husband isn't much of a dancer
so he just shuffled his feet as we rubbed our bodies together.

The champagne went straight to my head,
then to my pussy (is it okay if I say that?), making
me all itchy and needy. After a few hours of drinking and dancing, I all but dragged him back to our
room. He wasn't in a hurry, though. He slowly
undressed me, kissing every part from my ears to
my knees. I stretched out on the bed and he nib-
bled my toes and fingers.

Well, let me say by the time he climbed on top
of me, I was really really ready for him. He thrust
into me and then just fucked me, long and slow,
exactly the way I like it. I was torn between my
impatience and my enjoyment, but it didn't matter.
He was going to do it his way, no matter what I
wanted.

After long, slow lovemaking, suddenly he
pounded into me like there was no tomorrow and

I went off like a firecracker. I think that night the
earth moved . . . for both of us.

A forty-six-year-old man wrote:

This might seem selfish or something, but the only
way I can really have a perfect orgasm is with my
own hand. I've been masturbating for as long as I
can remember and I've perfected my release in a
way that no woman could ever duplicate.

It begins with a fantasy. Early on they were pretty
benign, but they've matured into something quite
kinky. I'm in an open field, naked. I can feel the grass
beneath my feet and the hot sun on my skin. I'm
sweating, but it's not from the heat of the day.

My heat comes from the fact that there's a
naked woman standing behind me with a strap-on
dildo firmly fastened around her hips. It has an
extension that she's inserted into her pussy so as
she fucks me, and I know she will, it will fuck her
too. She pushes on the small of my back to remind
me to bend over the fence that's just a foot in front
of me. I don't want her to do this, and yet I do.
The excitement is tremendous and my cock aches
from deep inside.

I look up and there are several men standing
around, watching, staring at my cock and at the
woman behind me. I turn so I can see her beautiful
breasts as she lubes my ass. I know it will hurt but I
also know that she's going to do it anyway. As she
slides the thick phallus into my rear, I rub my cock
with my slippery hand.

I come in the fantasy as I come in real life. The
orgasms aren't always perfect, but most come
close. Several have been as perfect as they can get.

A twenty-six-year-old woman wrote:

An old boyfriend of mine liked to play pretend games in the bedroom. One he made up really got to me and I think I had the perfect orgasm that night.

We walked into the bedroom one evening and he said, "Let's pretend this is a doctor's office and you're here for your annual checkup." I was game so I went along. I undressed and stretched out on the bed. He called me Ms. Smith.

"Ms. Smith," he said, "I need to do a breast exam first." He slowly kneaded my breasts and pulled at the nipples. There was something really erotic about the way he did it, so professional and uninvolved. It was incredibly kinky and got my pussy really wet. Happily he wasn't nearly finished yet.

"Now, Ms. Smith, I need you to put your heels up close to your butt so I can do the pelvic."

I thought I'd die from my excitement. I could hardly breathe as I raised my knees. As I lay there I was amazed to find he had a pair of rubber gloves like the ones in all the doctor movies. He pulled them on really slowly then slid his fingers through my pubic hair. "I'm sorry if this is a bit uncomfortable," he said, his voice still firm and unemotional. How he could stay so uninvolved I'll never know, but it was really like being part of a doctor's exam. Somehow I was a bit embarrassed to be so excited.

"My goodness, Ms. Smith," he said, sliding his fingers into me. "You're very wet. I hope this isn't arousing you. That wouldn't be a good idea here in the doctor's office."

That boyfriend knew me all too well so his words just made me hotter. Then he probed and poked, pressing on my belly as those fingers kept pushing and rubbing. "I have to test your clitoris," he said, stroking my hard clit with his free hand. Part of me didn't want to be excited and that was more exciting than anything. He continued to rub, keeping me just on the verge of climax, but never letting me over the edge.

One wet finger slid to my rear hole and, as he pushed it into me, he said, "Now for the rectal."

I came, hard. I couldn't help it. I spasmed and couldn't keep my hips still. I think I came for about half an hour, then collapsed from exhaustion. I think that was the most perfect orgasm I've ever had. Oh, and we made love several times that night so he had some pretty good ones too.

Okay, you get the idea. One writer said that it has to be part of a loving relationship; another had her perfect orgasm with a stranger, no love, just sex; yet another masturbates. One stated that he has to share it with his partner, while another wanted to just lie there and let his partner do everything. For one it was pretty much plain vanilla and for someone else it was the kinkiest night of her life.

So what should I do in a book called *The Perfect Orgasm*? I'm going to suggest how to give and get the building blocks—if we go back to my sandwich analogy, the bread, condiments, and sides. With those ingredients and your own desires, you can build your own perfect orgasm. As you read, you'll find lots of letters from real people who've found their paths to their perfect orgasm. There will be sections titled *How to Give It* and *How to Get It*. Of course, giving and getting are intermingled, so read it all.

Some of the blocks I discuss might not be ones you'd choose for your encounter, and that's fine. Everyone is different. One man might want tuna and pickles on a pita; another might want egg salad and chocolate sauce. If one section isn't your cup of tea, skip it and try another. But don't make the mistake of rejecting an idea because you think you're supposed to. Give anything that might appeal to you or your partner a chance. You never know.

What happens after you have the perfect orgasm? Does perfection mean that tomorrow's climax will fall short? Not on your life! Not only will you be able to build a perfect orgasm by the end of this book, but you'll have the tools to keep building new and different perfect orgasms for as long as you wish.

A few words about words. Throughout this book sexual acts are called both by their technical names and by the common slang that many folks use. Words like *pussy* and *cunt; cock, prick,* and *dick*; and *screwing* and *tit fucking* abound. Please try not to let the nouns and verbs obscure the message. If they offend you, I'm sorry. Try to get past them and find the ideas beneath.

Also, I frequently get into the gender thing. I tend to get buried in *he or she, him or her,* and so on. Sometimes I just give up and use one gender or the other. If the activity suits and you find you're reading the incorrect gender, just change it in your mind.

One more thing. This book is filled with letters from folks who wrote to my Web site. Many of the letters fit into several categories, so I made some pretty random decisions. I put them in the one that made the most sense at the time, but they might explain an activity or technique from another chapter. I also occasionally repeat myself in various chapters. For example you'll find information about lubricants and condoms in several sections. It's important to each and, since many folks will be skipping from chapter to chapter, I take no chances that important information might be missed. So let your fingers do the walking.

So . . . open your mind and relax. Let's begin at the start of the menu.

THE FOUNDATION

Chapter 1

COMMUNICATION

IF YOU AND YOUR PARTNER ARE ANYTHING LIKE Ed and me, you've gotten past any initial reluctance to discuss new things. *Bravo!* If that's the case you can probably skip this section. If, however, you're like the majority of couples in the world, there are things still left to try, and you're not particularly eager to bring up the subject even though your toes curl when you think about it. These things don't have to be monumental. Maybe it's playing in the hot tub, or doing it doggy-style. Or maybe it's something really off center, like anal sex or spanking. Wouldn't it be a shame if both of you had the same deliciously kinky thought but neither of you ever had the courage to say anything?

Scary, isn't it? Talking—or communicating in any way—about those "dirty little thoughts" that tease and titillate. Is there risk in letting your partner know about them? There might be, but it might be a risk well worth taking. I've gotten letters from so many people who, encouraged by contributors to my Web site, finally found a way to discuss their deepest desires with their partner, with orgasmic results.

The best way to move toward the perfect orgasm is to communicate your desires to your partner. Even now you have ideas about what you want but no idea how to tell your partner about them.

I know how communication goes—been there, done that. You finally work up the courage to tell him what you'd like to try. You begin. "Darling, I've been wanting to suggest something to add to our, uh, well, uh, our bedroom stuff."

At that moment you watch your partner's body language. His body stiffens, his arms and legs cross, and, although he is trying to keep trying to keep his face impassive, you sense a tightening around his eyes. You hesitate, then eventually you continue, "Never mind. What would you like for dinner?" He looks so relieved that you aren't having one of those conversations that you shove your desires to the back of your brain, never to be heard from again, except in your fantasies.

Maybe that's not your scenario. Here's another. You're in bed and she's touching you in the same old places in the same old way and, although you're getting turned on, you want something else. "Honey," you whisper.

She stops what she's doing and gets serious. "Yes, darling."

"Well, could you, I mean . . ." Again that tightening. Now you feel it in her hands and arms. Then you simply say, "I love you. Come here, baby."

Next, you try what's called mirroring. You do to him what you'd like him to do to you. You touch harder or softer and, although he moans and enjoys, he doesn't mirror what you're doing back. With a sigh, you resign yourself to the same ol' same ol'.

It doesn't have to be that way.

Okay, if you're so smart, Joan, how can I tell my partner what I want?

I've got several suggestions.

How to Get It

First, and foremost, your partner might be telling you things every time you make love. Be aware of his movements, his moans, his breathing. What turns him on? Specifically. Does playing with your nipples make him hot? Have you ever played with his? Does he seem to want it slower or faster? Tune yourself in to him for an evening. You'll be amazed at what you can learn.

Now return the favor. Show him with your breathing, movements, and moans what you like. He wasn't born knowing any more than you were. You have to help him, teach him what you like, especially if you can't tell him just yet.

Making noise during sex is a great way to improve things. If you're a moaner, your partner should quickly learn that the volume is an indicator of how good things are. If he presses harder, you moan louder (or stop moaning), which tells him how you like to be touched. If you wiggle, toward or away, it's another way of showing him what you like.

If you decide to be a bit more verbal, always be positive. Let's say you want her to touch you differently—softer, harder, longer, shorter, whatever. I know you don't want to say, *I don't enjoy what you're doing, do it this way.*

Try saying, "I love it when you . . ." or "Softer touches make me so hot . . ." or "Ooo, do more of that." There are so many ways to couch suggestions in a positive light that will not only tell her what you want, but also reinforce how wonderful her lovemaking is.

If you want to make love in a different place or at a different time, do it. I know that he usually initiates sex, but there's no law against you doing it from time to time. Jump his bones. Grab his crotch. Be aggressive. He'll probably be surprised, but he'll also be delighted that you've taken the initiative. Maybe it's just lighting the candles. Be brave. It will be well worth your while.

There are more ways of subtle communication, especially if

you're relatively new to a relationship. You can mention things you *don't* like—in the abstract and not during lovemaking, of course, but before or after. "I'm not particularly fond of making love on the floor, even if it is in front of a roaring fire. I tried it once and got rug burns on my butt." Silly little bit of stuff, but it lightens the moment and invites your partner to open up a bit; it might eventually lead to comments on what he does like.

A way to communicate without words is to take his hand, or whatever part of his anatomy you're trying to alter, and move it. Place your hand over his and show him what you want. Lighter touches, touches in a slightly different place. Remember, he's trying to learn about you just as much as you're trying to learn about him. Every woman (and man) is different. If you're new to the relationship, he is probably trying to learn what you like. If you take the first step and help him learn, maybe he'll tell you some of the things you need to know about pleasing him.

If your relationship is long standing, he's probably slipped into what we all do, habit. Familiarity is nice, but sometimes you want something different. Again, use your hands to show him what you want.

If your partner guides your hand, take it as a compliment. It is. He's telling you ways to make your lovemaking even better, and isn't that what you want?

Okay. Now you've gotten braver and you want to actually talk about sex. It is said that men communicate best when sitting side by side, while women do best face to face. Since it's usually the man who has more difficulty talking about these risky topics, lying on the bed, holding hands, might work best. You can also try sitting on the sofa, and when he stares into space instead of looking into your eyes, let him.

Another way to ask for something you want is a technique I invented called bookmarking. It involves using stories, articles, or what have you from any source. Since you have this book in your hands, let's use it as an example.

6

First you read. Lots. Find out what's out there and try to ascertain what, exactly, curls your toes; what you want in the bedroom. I'm not talking generalizations. "I want more romance." "I want more foreplay." "I want him to be more creative." Those aren't specific enough. Go for things like, "I want him to suck on my breasts." "I want to play doctor." "I want to make love in the morning instead of at night." "I want lovemaking to last longer than it does now."

Now let's say you've narrowed it down to a few things to start with. Don't try to take giant leaps. Small steps will work better, and you'll see rewards more quickly.

Okay, back to bookmarking.

Find a story in this book (or elsewhere) that illustrates something you want to try. Put a bookmark into the story and give it to your partner to read in private. That way he can get past the knee-jerk *She isn't happy with my lovemaking* reaction. If you're worried that he won't understand the purpose of your bookmark, give him these pages to read.

Guys, if you get a bookmarked story, she's not telling you something bad at all. She's trying to find ways to make sex still better. Let go of the natural resistance and think a bit about what she's saying. She's telling you that she doesn't want anyone else, just you. And she wants you two to have more fun making love with each other.

If you find the idea that she's suggested intriguing, great. You've found something you two agree on. Later in this book you two will find lots of concrete ways to make it all happen. For now you've communicated. She's made a suggestion, and you've allowed as how it might be fun. *Bravo!*

But what if you don't like the idea she's indicated? *Slow-dancing? Not my thing. Spanking? Never happen in this life!* That's okay, too. At least you two have taken the first step. Maybe she's suggested morning lovemaking and the thought of doing anything before you have your coffee is anathema. Fine, that's your choice. Read through this book or find a story on the Net or browse whatever material you can find and give her a bookmarked passage.

It might take several exchanges of bookmarks, but eventually you'll come up with something that both of you want to try. *Bravo!*

A variation on the idea of bookmarking is telling stories in the dark. Have you ever tried telling stories in the dark? Why in the dark? That way you don't have to look at each other, so it's less embarrassing. Begin lying in bed, horny and ready for lovemaking. Then start a sexy story with the kind of setup you might read in a novel. "I've always fantasized about being caught in a ski cabin with the snow falling outside, a big fire in the fireplace, a soft furry rug, you and me. We'd . . ."—I leave the rest to you. In the story you can mention things you've always wanted to play with: oral sex, spanking, whatever you've always dreamed of. Remember, right now it's just a story, not a confession.

Hold hands while telling stories and put your other hand on his chest. You might well be able to feel his reaction to the activity you just talked about. Do his muscles tighten or his fingers clench? What does that mean? Is it a good reaction, something he'd like to try but is too embarrassed to mention, or a bad one, something so unpleasant you'd better steer the story in another direction? I'm sure you'll find out within the next few moments, and it will be a great piece of information.

Another way to find out what he likes is to stop the story and suggest that he pick it up. Maybe, in the story, you're straddling him. "What would you like me to do now?" Then listen very carefully to what he suggests. He's telling you his desires. Store that information away, and then encourage him. "That sounds so sexy." You can even do what he's suggesting right then and there.

Here are a few ideas for story starters in case you can't come up with any on your own:

- It's their wedding night and he's quite experienced. She's a virgin.

- He's a customer and she's a professional.

- She's his boss so he has to do everything she says, after hours.

- She is skinny-dipping alone and is caught by a hunky lifeguard.

- He's in the slave market and sees her up for sale.

- He's a spy and she's saved him from the bad guys, for now. They might only have one night together.

- He's bought up her father's gambling debts so she'd better be nice to him.

- She's a police officer who's pulled him over for speeding. He'll do anything to avoid getting a ticket.

Be brave. The rewards can be greater than you ever dreamed.

Chapter 2

ORGASMS

WHAT IS AN ORGASM? THE ANSWER SOUNDS pretty obvious, and for a man, it is. According to the *Random House Dictionary of the English Language,* an orgasm is "the physical and emotional sensation experienced at the culmination of a sexual act, as intercourse or masturbation, being a result of stimulation of the sexual organs, and typically followed in the male by ejaculation."

Phew. Sounds pretty dull. If you read the definition, ladies, you will realize that, although orgasm is pretty well marked for a man—ejaculation—it's a bit hazy for a woman. Are those spasms we wait for necessary for an "orgasm"? Is the feeling of contentment and fulfillment that most of us get after lovemaking even when no fireworks have exploded orgasm too? Who knows and who cares? What we're aiming for is great sex, sex that leaves us—men and women—feeling complete and somehow finished, satisfied.

To build a great (and maybe perfect) orgasm, you have to start with a few basics: the foundation. There are several issues, applicable to different segments of the population. Let's begin with the predictability of your old habits, as well as what to do about privacy, space, the kids, birth control, and condoms.

Predictability

This section is for those who've been with the same partner for a while and whose lovemaking has fallen into a pattern. It begins with the same signals. You know the ones—he climbs into bed, rolls over, and kisses you in that special way that says, *Baby, let's.* Or he lights the candles in the bedroom, or he comes to bed without his pajama bottoms.

She's not immune to the nudge-nudge-wink-wink either. She wears that nightie that he likes, rolls over and cuddles against his back, reaches around and strokes his belly.

Then lovemaking takes the same path. It might have been a delicious path several dozen trips before, but by now it's become a habit, maybe even a rut. There's nothing wrong with that, and if that's what does it for you, great. I suspect, however, if you're reading this book, that you want something different, something that will bring you closer to your idea of the perfect orgasm.

How to Give It

Do something daring. Try whispering something sexy in your partner's ear at a party when he can't do anything about it right then. "I want your body." "I've got a little surprise for you when we get home." How daring can you be? Can you grab his crotch when no one can see? Can you bite her ear or nibble her neck? Why the heck not?

More daring? How about arriving for dinner at the boss's house and, just before you ring the doorbell, telling your partner you've forgotten to put on your undies? Or making an audiotape for your lover to play in the car on the way home that describes all the naughty things you've got planned? Print a picture of what you want to do later from a Web site and hide it in her briefcase.

How to Shake Things Up

Where to start? How about changing your scent? The sense of smell triggers memories and feelings more than any other, so use that. Change your perfume, your shampoo, your body wash. Slather on body lotion with a new aroma—spicy if you're always floral or musky, whatever. Guys, use that bottle of cologne that's been sitting in the back of your medicine chest since your mother-in-law got it for you for Christmas several years ago.

If your partner always initiates lovemaking, make the first move yourself. Begin with "Honey" in that tone that says it all, or "Wanna fool around?" Put a sexy CD on the player, maybe slow-dance music or something from when you were dating. Light candles in the bedroom, or leave the lights on when you climb into bed (or turn them off—whatever's different). Wear a sexy new bra or a pair of satin boxers to remind both of you of the lovemaking to come. Go to bed nude, or wear a pretty new nightie or a pajama top or bottom if you usually sleep raw. Take an old T-shirt and cut holes in strategic places.

Kiss good night with your eyes open and suggest that your lover do the same. Use your hands—knead his buttocks or caress her cheeks. Comb your fingers through your partner's hair.

There are usually ideas in every issue of women's magazines, but nothing is going to happen unless you gather your courage and do something. That's all. Gather your courage, take the risk, and *do something!*

Finding Quiet Time

This next section is for folks with children. Again, if that's not you, skip on, or read anyway. You never know what life has in store.

Kids are wonderful little people, and many couples have them running around. They are a joy and a delight, except when you and your partner are trying to create or maintain a good sex life. Then they can really be murder, especially when you're trying something new. Been there, done that, in spades!

The problem is twofold. At the end of the day you're both too pooped to participate; also, you worry that Junior will wander into the bedroom at just the wrong moment.

I had a friend many years ago who, as a child, had a glow-in-the-dark religious picture beside her bed. One night, at age four or so, she decided to give her parents a visitation, so she held the picture over the lamp beside her bed until it was glowing brightly. Then, carrying it over her head, she walked into her parents' bedroom. Well, they had a visitation all right . . . Need I say more? In later years it became a delicious family anecdote. At the time it happened, though, I can imagine that the parents decided to swear off sex for quite a while.

Let's get practical. You can't move toward the perfect orgasm without private time. Here are a few tips.

How to Get It

If your kids are old enough, get them in the habit of respecting your quiet time. Explain that Mommy and Daddy are having private time (or whatever you want to call it), and as long as the door is closed, they must stay away. If they really need something, tell them to knock and wait to be told to come in. By the way, you should respect their privacy as well.

If your children are too young to understand, get a lock for your bedroom door. Never lock kids in their rooms; just lock them out of yours. The easiest way is to get an old-fashioned hook and eye, and mount it as high as you can reach to prevent the little ones from accidentally locking it themselves.

But how can I do that? My child sleeps in my room from time to time. I don't want little Johnny or Janie to think I don't love him or her anymore.

Having Junior sleep in your bed is a really bad idea. For years child psychologists have said that kids should have their own room, or at least an area to sleep in that is theirs. Of course I can't help you rearrange your house, but I can help you make the break.

Let's assume that the little one is a boy, just to get around my perpetual s/he dilemma. *How do I get my son to sleep in his own room? As the commercials say, Just do it. But he'll scream.* Yup. Little Johnny will scream bloody murder for as much as several nights running until you're ready to scream yourself. Make the resolve and stick to it. It just has to be. Here are a few ways to lessen the impact.

Pick a time when you can afford to lose a little sleep, maybe by beginning on a Friday night. Then discuss with the child (if he is old enough) that you and Daddy need your own space, and the little darling will have his as well. Maybe he can help decorate the room. Let him pick out new sheets or a new sleeping bag and reward him with a new toy or game. Get him a flashlight that he can sleep with and turn on anytime he feels alone. When he's tired, hug him and put him to bed in his room. Make sure he has a glass of water and whatever else he might need. Then go into your room, close the door, and wait.

Will he get up? Of course. And bang on your door? Yup. Scream? Probably. When he does, tell him firmly that he has his own room and it's time for him to settle down. Will he go? Probably not. So hunker down and reassure him, but don't let him in. If it makes you more comfortable, lead him back to bed and tuck him in with a kiss and his flashlight. But be prepared. This might go on for a while.

Maybe you'll be lucky and he'll settle down and fall asleep. Okay, it might take several nights, but I can assure you that eventually he'll get the idea. You might want to make a little fuss the first morning he doesn't get up. Reward him with a big hug and something special for breakfast. Oh, and now that you've done it, don't backslide. Don't decide that he's used to it now, so you can let him stay in your room once in a while. You'll end up going through the same pain yet again.

Get Out of the House

If you can't get any real privacy at home, or even just for the heck of it, it's time for the Notell Motel. Why? In your house, you're Mommy and Daddy instead of the lovers you were before the kids were born.

That sounds easy, but I know all too well that it's not. How can you possibly manage it? First, get a babysitter who can give you several hours of private time. It doesn't have to be all night, of course, but that would be the ideal. If money is a problem, call on the grandparents or other relatives. Make a deal with some friends whose kids are about your own children's ages, agreeing to watch their kids overnight in exchange for watching yours. The pain of having the neighbor's kids for a night will be more than outweighed by the joy of having an entire night to yourselves.

Now that you've gotten some time, don't decide to spend it sleeping or doing some activity that doesn't get you two interacting, like going to a movie or watching TV. Talk. You remember talking. Talk about things that don't involve household maintenance or toilet training. Talking involves discussing each other and what's important to each of you. Intimacy. Remember that?

If you can, make a reservation for a nice relaxing dinner and an hour or two (or all night if you're lucky) at a motel. Then spend some time recalling your first dates and the first time you made love: the wonderful heat, the closeness, maybe even the embarrassments. Giggle. It's good for the soul and for the next step down the path toward the perfect orgasm.

Timing

How long do you want your perfect lovemaking to last? Most say it depends on the mood. "Sometimes I like lovely, luxurious sex, with lots of stroking and cuddling, long foreplay, and teasing," one woman wrote. "At times I want it short and hard," another said. A letter from a third stated, "I hate to admit it, but sometimes I want a quickie. Is that bad?"

What actually is a quickie? Here's how I define it: In the good sense, it's a brief encounter with both parties heated up long before they actually get together so they are ready for intercourse almost immediately. Then they come together in a great rush, fucking fast and furious until both are satisfied.

In the bad sense, a quickie is a sexual encounter that leaves one partner dissatisfied. The former is delicious occasionally; the latter is to be avoided. Let's deal with the negative connotation.

How to Get Past the Quickie

I guess this section is more about what to do about it. If it's okay with you that your partner occasionally climaxes and leaves you hanging, great. If, however, there are times when you want more, ask for it. It's really important. Don't lie there and make him (let's assume it's a him who has ejaculated and rolled over) guess or play the martyr. Ask for what you want.

Be specific. Don't say, *I want more loving.* Rather, say, "Baby, please touch me. I'm still excited and I know you can help." Put his hand where you want it to be. Be aggressive with him. If he's already come, climb on top of him and rub your genitals on his hip. Please yourself; he just pleased himself.

You can also try to slow him down. Say "Don't come yet," with lots of heavy breathing. "I need you. Wait for me." Your orgasm, perfect or otherwise, is your responsibility too, not just his.

A forty-eight-year-old woman wrote:

> Sometimes my husband loves a quickie but when he does it that way I'm left so hungry that I go into the bathroom and masturbate until I'm satisfied. Recently I decided that bathroom pleasure isn't enough for me anymore. Last week he did his usual fuck and roll. I was just about ready to come so I walked around to his side of the bed, climbed in, and straddled his face.
>
> He loves giving me oral sex and he's really good at it. He got the message really quickly and used his tongue and hands to help me over the edge. Later, we talked and he told me that I could say, "Wait a minute" and he would. With a laugh he said he couldn't wait too long, but he agreed that if I wanted more he would help me afterward.

A thirty-nine-year-old woman wrote:

> My husband and I used to have a problem with quickies. Now we use that word as a cue so I can tell him that he's rushing me. When I say, "No quickies tonight," he realizes that I would like him to slow down. He usually does. When he can't, he uses his fingers and my trusty vibrator to get me off.

Birth Control

Another topic that needs addressing is birth control. If this goes against your beliefs, skip this section.

Pills and other hormonal contraceptives, diaphragms, intrauterine devices (IUDs), sponges, and more work with varying degrees of dependability. I suggest that you seek serious advice from your doctor before deciding on the method that works for both of you.

I remember almost forty years ago, after the birth of my second child, I wanted to obtain birth control pills, a new method for me. My then-husband was in the military and I knew the army hospital wouldn't dispense "the pill," so I telephoned a gynecologist recommended by a woman in my apartment complex. When I discussed my problem with the nurse who answered the phone, her voice turned cold and she said, "Madam, that won't be possible. Doctor is Catholic." Needless to say, I found another physician. Lesson? Find someone to talk to who can answer all your questions and make serious suggestions.

Life is so much easier now. There are lots of methods of birth control for long-term couples. Neither pills and other hormone regulation methods nor IUDs need thought prior to intercourse. For those who want the ultimate in spontaneity, those are probably best.

There are sponges, spermicides, and diaphragms, which must be used within hours of lovemaking. A word of advice. I used a diaphragm for many years with perfect results. To keep lovemaking spontaneous, I inserted the diaphragm every night. That way I didn't have to groan and climb out of bed at the wrong moment.

There are surgical procedures, such as tubal ligations and vasectomies, that can prevent pregnancy. With these procedures, however, reversibility is not a sure thing by any means; it's a permanent and final decision for most couples. It's certainly up to you and your partner which method works best for you, and some research might help you discuss the issue. Once you've come to an agreement, a doctor's visit is a starting point.

Every method has a certain pregnancy risk factor, although most are quite low. Most methods work fine for most people, but each can have its drawbacks. Some women find there are libido issues with hormones, while others have gotten pregnant despite an IUD or diaphragm.

A word about playing pregnancy roulette. Many couples try the withdrawal method, pulling the penis out of the vagina prior to ejaculation, and believe it's birth control. It isn't. Pre-cum, that thick fluid that leaks from the penis before climax, is filled with sperm, and yes, you most certainly can become pregnant from just that. Likewise, the rhythm method—trying to find the specific times of the month when she's not fertile—isn't reliable either. We used to tease that people who use the rhythm method are called parents. It doesn't work well enough to depend on it since women can become pregnant at different times in their cycle. There are even women who can become pregnant while they have their period.

Condoms

Condoms are the main method of birth control for a large number of couples, both those in long-term relationships and those looking for short-term companionship. If used correctly, they can prevent pregnancy almost 100 percent of the time and are the only way to protect yourself from the dangers of disease. If you're new to a committed relationship, I also suggest that both of you get an AIDS test just to be on the safe side.

Condoms must be used properly if they are to do their job. They must be unrolled over the entire penis prior to *any* penis–vagina contact and kept in place until intercourse is completed. When unrolled, a condom should have a reservoir at the tip, a space for fluids so they aren't forced up the shaft and out the top. Then, after intercourse, one of you has to hold the latex during withdrawal to keep all semen contained.

Latex condoms are the only kind that protect from disease transmission. Natural skins can keep sperm under control, but viruses go right through the microscopic holes.

If you use any type of artificial lubrication with the condoms, the lube must be water-soluble. Petroleum products such as baby oil and Vaseline can eat away at the latex and create tiny holes that let both sperm and viruses pass through. Purchase K-Y Jelly, Astroglide, or one of the many other available water-based lubricants at your local store, a catalog, or an adult Web site. Remember to only use a water-soluble lube. There are also combination lubricants and spermicides that both provide lubrication and prevent conception.

Condoms come in sizes. Most of those sold in neighborhood stores are of the one-size-fits-most variety, but if you're particularly small or particularly large, check around for the correct size. Web sites that sell adult products have lots of different kinds. Don't, however, decide that it's a status thing to be a "big guy" and insist on large-size condoms. If a condom doesn't fit properly, it won't do its job and might slip off.

Take care with that one in your wallet. If it's been there more than a few months or has passed the expiration date, replace it. Condoms become brittle and can crack during use. Ladies, always carry several yourself so you don't succumb to the heat of the moment. No bareback riding. Ever!

One last thing. This might sound ridiculous, but don't reuse a condom. Folks have been known to do that, particularly if they are someplace where condoms aren't available.

Okay, I can hear you now. *I don't want to use those things.* Too bad. You have to if you're going to prevent disease and pregnancy. You can, however, make using a condom more fun or at least less odious.

Using Condoms Made Easier

First, select fun condoms. There are lots of sites on the Net that sell silly (but useful) condoms. Get some in different colors or ones that glow in the dark. Find some with pictures on them, or with flavored lubricants. Try the textured kind and see whether she can feel the difference. Next time you use one, turn it inside out and see whether he can feel it.

Make putting one on part of your lovemaking routine. Let her help. Slowly. It's really not such a chore.

I hate the way they dull the sensation. I can sympathize with your reluctance, but using a condom isn't a matter of choice. Take a lot of time during foreplay to get penile stimulation. Show her how to stroke you, rub your cock between her breasts, masturbate while she watches. By the time you put the condom on, it won't feel like as much of a letdown.

A word about oral sex and condoms. Many scientists think that unprotected oral sex is a high-risk activity, and so there are products to protect you from the danger of infection during oral play. I don't know whether those scientists are right, so a word to the wise should suffice.

A *twenty-seven-year-old woman wrote:*

Try this one on your lover: My boyfriend and I were making love, and as part of the process, he asked me to slip a condom on his shaft. I guess I was feeling pretty naughty and I wanted to tease him a bit.

I got a condom from my nightstand drawer then slowly opened the package and took it out—in slow motion. I took his cock in my mouth and started to tease him with my tongue around the head and then his slit. I sat back, put the condom on the head of his cock, rolled it down just one turn and then started licking the length of his cock moving counterclockwise.

I could tell that he liked what I was doing from the comments he was making. I then unrolled the condom one more turn and teased his balls with my tongue. Then I unrolled the condom yet one more turn, while I teased his cock by licking the uncovered shaft.

I continued that action—teasing either his cock or balls, then rolling the condom an additional turn—until his dick was completely covered. As one last cock teaser I flicked my tongue around him at the base of his cock while I cupped and lightly squeezed his balls. At this point he begged me to make love to him—he was actually screaming—so I mounted and rode him to a mutual orgasm. It didn't take long!

A forty-year-old man wrote:

My wife and I still use condoms as our primary method of birth control but it's not really a problem. My wife is a wicked tease and, as she puts it on me, she keeps stroking me and asking, "Should I unroll more?" I can never decide on the answer—do I want her to unroll it so we can have intercourse or do I want her to keep stroking me.

Ahhhh. Decisions.

A thirty-six-year-old man wrote:

I was once with a new partner and we both knew that condoms were a must. We had been kissing and fondling each other when she asked me to change the CD on the stereo in the motel room. I got up and put in new music while she lit some candles and turned off the lights in the room. I was just getting ready to get in bed when she said, "Stay right there!" With that she knelt down in front of me and began to play with me, cupping my balls with one hand as she ran her other up and down my cock. She then took my cock into her mouth and went down on the shaft as far as possible. My cock, which had been erect, was even more so now and it strained upward.

"I want to make love with you," I said. She looked up at me and smiled, then continued to play with my shaft and balls. I was in heaven, enjoying the sensations of her hands stroking my cock. Finally I could stand it no longer. "I want you now," I said.

"I want you too," she said, and got on the bed. As I moved to enter her, I happened to look at my cock. She had managed to slip a condom on and unroll it without my knowing it.

A thirty-seven-year-old woman wrote:
Putting on a condom isn't very sexy, so to make that action seem less of a chore I keep a variety of condoms, colored (I love the black ones), ribbed, studded, and even glow in the dark ones, in my nightstand drawer. As part of foreplay, I guess, we sit and carefully select the one we'll use each night.

A forty-year-old woman wrote:
One thing my husband and I do to make condoms work for us is to pour some lubricant (we use Astroglide) inside the condom before I roll it down on his erection. It gives a slippery feeling and it's also good just for hand jobs. It doesn't feel as rough and gives that wet feel that women have. My husband loves it.

Note: Take care that the lube doesn't make the

condom so slippery that it slides off during love-making, defeating the entire purpose.

A twenty-eight-year-old man wrote:

I knew a woman once who could put a condom on me with her mouth. It might take a bit of practice for others to master the technique but it's sure fun learning.

THE FILLING

Chapter 3

ANTICIPATION

ORGASMS DON'T JUST HAPPEN; THEY NEED TIME and buildup. It is said that man flames like a match while woman heats like an iron. Anticipation, playing, taking time to let her get as hot as she can—all can make the path toward the perfect orgasm longer, yet more satisfying.

A thirty-one-year-old woman wrote:

You asked about the perfect orgasm. This may sound strange but although my husband and I have had a lot of great orgasms I don't want to label any of them perfect. I want to keep trying (evil grin). I do remember one in particular.

Let me say that sometimes Mike's pleasure is enough for me, and I don't have to actually come. It takes me a long time to get hot enough and occasionally, okay maybe more than just occasionally, he comes before I'm really ready.

I remember once, when we were still dating, we never made it back to his dorm room. We went to a movie we'd been wanting to see, only to discover very quickly that, despite the hype, the film was dreadful. We considered leaving, but I guess he was in the mood to neck and to hell with what was on the screen. The film had a lot of R-rated sex, lots of heavy breathing, moaning and such, and I guess it got Mike in the mood. We started to make out like the horny college kids we used to be. It was such a gas, being there in the dark theater, knowing that we had to be quiet while we fooled around. Since we couldn't actually do it there in the multiplex we teased for about an hour. I was wearing a blouse that opened down the front so he had me all unbuttoned and was kissing and licking my breasts. It drives me crazy when he flicks his tongue over my nipples. The air-conditioning was on high in the theater so my tits got really cold where he'd been licking and my nipples got really tight. It made Mike crazy.

I had stopped paying any attention to the film so when Mike's hand started to slither up my thigh I could concentrate on how good and exciting it was. He played with my crotch through my jeans until I was so hot and so wet I thought I'd come right there. We didn't even notice that the movie had ended until the lights came up and all the people started to leave. I quickly buttoned my blouse and we hustled to the car.

It was after eleven, so we drove to a dark corner of the theater's parking lot, unable to wait any longer. Without a word, we shifted to the backseat and he was all over me, pulling at my clothes and his. He was inside me fast, banging away. Usually I want his hands on me, his fingers inside me, but this time he just slammed his dick into me and I came. Just like that. Maybe it was all the playing beforehand, I don't know. I do know that when his big dick rammed into me I went off. I don't think I'll ever forget that night.

A forty-two-year-old man wrote:

The best orgasm I can remember isn't one of mine, but one of my wife's. It started the evening of my company New Year's Eve party. My wife, Michelle, was wearing a little blue dress that I think she must have bought merely to drive me crazy. It was low cut—not so low that everyone else got a view but low enough that when we walked side by side I could see down between her gorgeous tits. The white lace at the tops of her bra cups made my palms itch. The dress had a swishy little skirt and flicked over her ass and her stockings and cute red high heels made her look like my personal hooker. Don't get me wrong, the dress was perfect for the party and, except in my mind, demure enough for the occasion.

Anyway, the party was at a club in the heart of the city. The food was great, the music loud, and the conversations interesting. As the evening wore on, lots of couples used the small dance floor, waiting for midnight. Michelle and I danced a lot, fast stuff where I could watch her move, and slow stuff so I could hold her and rub my body against hers. I could feel her nipples getting hard and I snuck a pinch whenever I thought I could do so without anyone seeing.

As the countdown to midnight began, everyone turned toward the DJ and screamed "One Minute to Go." Michelle moved so her back was against my chest. I wrapped one arm around her ribs, my thumb rubbing the side of her breast. Usually Michelle was a calm, quiet lover, but that night something got into her and she let me do things I'd never have considered trying before. I could feel her purring against my chest. God, she was hot.

I don't know what possessed me, but I lifted the back of her skirt and, looking totally innocent, slid my hand up the back of one thigh until I found the top of her stocking. Above, that's the softest place I know, the few inches of skin between the stocking and her panties, so I stroked. And as I stroked I felt her tremble.

"Thirty Seconds." Her panties were so wet that I couldn't resist rubbing. I had to bend my knees a bit but I managed to slide my fingers toward the front of the crotch of her panties. I couldn't believe it when she moved her feet to part her thighs. I found her swollen clit and rhythmically rubbed, using my other arm to brace her so she didn't fall. At "Fifteen Seconds" everyone started to count down and I rubbed in rhythm to their counting. For some silly reason I wanted her to come right at midnight.

Michelle and I had been married for three years at that point and making love for several years before that so I knew her body pretty well. I leaned down and told her that she was going to come right at zero, then bit her ear, breathing hot and heavy. "Five, Four, Three"—I felt her body stiffen. "Two, One." "Baby," I whispered, "come now."

"Happy New Year!" She came. I could feel her body jerk and quickly turned her and covered her mouth with mine so she wouldn't scream. I found her pussy beneath the front of that little skirt and slipped my fingers inside her to help her finish.

Later, she was limp and I guided her from the dance floor to one of the little tables. She told me that nothing like that had ever happened before. We've become more adventurous lovers since and we've had lots of orgasms. That one, however, is the one I remember most, the most perfect orgasm I've ever given.

You might have noticed that both these letters revolve around situations during which the couple couldn't have intercourse right away. Anticipation. Teasing and playing. So many of us have forgotten to wait, to let it simmer, the way we used to. So how do we get it back?

Let's say you're going out with your husband or wife and you want your partner's thoughts to revolve around hot sex all evening. Maybe you're going somewhere with the kids, or friends, or other folks around, however, so you've got to be very secret.

How to Give It for Her

Tell him what's on your mind just before you leave. "Honey, I just want to mention that I bought a new black teddy to wear later." If you want, sometime during the evening, remove your bra, then brush your now naked-beneath-your-clothes breasts against him so he knows what you've done. Showing, in this case, is so much better than just telling.

Scratch the back of his neck as you pass behind him, or, if you've got enough privacy, grab his ass. It's so unladylike, and so provocative.

How to Give It for Him

Just before you leave, tell the babysitter that you'll be late getting home. If you can, make a reservation at the Notell Motel for after the normal end of the evening. Even if you stay just an hour, it will be worth it. Oh, and make sure she knows your plans.

Remember, you can still do it in the car on the way home. Stop at a quiet spot or even in your own driveway. It will be really awkward and lots of fun.

If you're in a public place, whisper a key word or phrase into her ear that will tell her you're thinking about the sex to come. It can be something simple like "Later, baby," or kinky like "Wanna fuck, lady?" Keep it within your comfort zone, but do it.

To build the excitement throughout the day, try leaving suggestive phone messages or e-mails for your lover. Just take care that she will be alone when she gets them. Slip a sexy note or story into your partner's briefcase or just hand him a flower with a red ribbon around the stem as you leave for work. Buy your lover a new pair of panties or briefs, something totally different from the usual. Then every movement will be a reminder of the evening to come.

A fifty-two-year-old man wrote:
> My idea of a perfect orgasm comes at the end of
> an evening of lots of teasing. I love loooooong
> foreplay and being that I am a guy this is probably
> unusual. My idea of great foreplay is an almost
> entire evening of teasing each other, and it needs
> to take place in public so you can't "do" each other.

Getting dressed up and going out to dinner is a good starting place for my wife and me. The rules? No underwear allowed, loose pants for me and she usually wears something teasing and sexy—maybe a short skirt and a top that shows a lot of cleavage. I love one particular top she wears. When she bends over I can see all the way down to her nipples.

While we are waiting to be seated at the restaurant my wife does that Sharon Stone cross-the-legs routine while other people are present or she bends over to fix her shoes so I get a good view. During dinner we give each other shoeless "crotch footsies" (which is why I wear baggy pants). Her gifted foot can really move my cock around much better when I wear looser clothing. While she's doing that, my foot can go all the way up her leg and tickle her cunt.

Sometimes we eat at a restaurant in the mall, then go to the lingerie store where we talk about what we want to buy, then wander to the adult toy store to look at all the dildos, cock rings, and other playthings. By then things are always really hot. Sometimes we make out in the car, and at others we nail each other as soon as we get home, right on the living room floor.

Foreplay

A thirty-three-year-old man wrote:
For me a long slow massage of a woman's body, exploring every little detail and being aware of

what makes her squirm and shiver, is the best way to get to the perfect orgasm for her and for me. I explore and keep doing everything she enjoys until she has an orgasm or two. I love touching her, stroking her, and knowing that what I'm doing is driving her crazy. I hold out until I'm ready to come, then fuck her wildly. It's so fabulous.

A forty-three-year-old woman wrote:

I'm a very sensual person, and sometimes I think sensuality is left out in foreplay. My ex-lover and I had a wonderful sex life, in part because of the foreplay. Sometimes we would take hours just touching each other and kissing passionately.

Most people kiss with eyes closed; it seems to be a natural reaction. During one of these times I suggested that we keep our eyes open as we kiss. At first it was a strange sensation, but quickly it became very exciting. No matter where I was kissing, nibbling, gently biting, I looked at him the whole time and he did the same. It was wonderful. We watched the excitement build in each other's eyes, which in turn made us more excited.

There are some positions that just don't allow that, of course, and for those we found that a mirror helps. We have a wide one over the dresser and a tall one on the back of the closet door. One is always in view.

They say the eyes are the window to the soul, and I tend to believe that. Give it a try, it's very sensual, erotic, and exciting.

Anticipation

A twenty-six-year-old woman wrote:

I am a twenty-six-year-old female but don't let the age fool you. I love long, erotic teasing sessions so much that I've developed foreplay to a fine art.

One place I enjoy erotic foreplay is in a semi-public try-on room at a place like Victoria's Secret. I like to select some sexy panties or even a bra then invite my current lover into the tiny room to get his opinion. He always likes what I've selected, of course.

Then I change into the next outfit. Since these rooms are really small I frequently have to rub my half-naked body against him while slipping on the next piece of sexy lingerie. This time I usually ask him to buckle the clasp on the bra or help me put the panties on. He's still completely dressed and can't really do the dirty deed right there since there's no real privacy. But doing anything like this in public where you might get caught is always exciting. I've suggested this little game to lots of my friends, and no one has ever come back with anything less than raves.

A sixty-year-old man wrote:

Call me old fashioned, but for me great sex always starts with great foreplay, and ballroom dancing is a great place to start. At a party with lots of people around a lady is quite sure that nothing's going to happen in full view of everyone else, so that gently stroking her back and caressing her hand doesn't cause any problem, even on a first date.

Dancing like this is just a way of touching and holding her in an allowable way, so that she gets used to you. Maybe later, when you're alone, she'll want another dance and after a while you can lead her into the bedroom. Dancing is also a way to get to know shy girls (and there are still lots around). Perhaps your date has never waltzed before. Showing her how is one way to let her see how considerate and gentle you are.

For long-term partners, showing off on the dance floor gives the lady confidence in your affection. It demonstrates that, if you dance well together, then there are a lot of more intimate things that you'll do well together too. Maybe it's bragging but I think other folks look at dancers and think about how good they must be in the bedroom.

That's my idea of the beginning of foreplay; couples of today's generation never even seem to hold hands, especially at discos and in clubs. They don't know what they're missing!

A fifty-two-year-old man wrote:
A perfect orgasm begins with long foreplay. I am dating a lady who is in her midfifties. We had slept together four times when she told me she liked and needed more foreplay. I was glad she broke through and told me this, even though I was a little uneasy at first since I've never played much with any lady before.

Grateful that she was so up-front about it, I thought about foreplay for a while and eventually came up with an idea. The next time we were together, I suggested that we sit across from each other at the kitchen table—naked! It was dynamite. We sipped Cognac and talked. I stared at her breasts frequently and she took some peeks at me, too. She got a long peek as I walked over to refill my glass with a full hard-on. After about twenty minutes she said, "I've had enough foreplay," and we ran to the bedroom for some great sex.

Since then we often sit naked or half naked having coffee or a drink, but although there is still a warm feeling, it doesn't have the same intense effect that it did that first time.

About Breasts and Nipples

Breasts play a tremendous part in sexuality and are an important landmark on the path toward the perfect orgasm. Large or small, women's breasts have been a fixation for men—and women too—since Og ogled Nog's breasts in the back of the cave.

Before I talk about women's breasts, however, let's dwell a moment on men's. Are they as sensitive as a woman's? Not usually. For many men, however, their nipples become as erect as a woman's and they enjoy having them played with as much as their female counterparts.

How to Give It for Her

A fifty-two-year-old man wrote:
It's only been in the last five years or so that my wife of twenty-six years has realized that my nipples

are really sensitive and tweaking them is guaranteed to get my cock erect. The first time she pinched me I thought I'd go through the ceiling—quite a discovery for both of us.

I've always played with her large nipples and she always enjoys it, but now she knows that I like it too. I really get hot when she sucks on them. It's taken some years, but mutual attention to this sensitive part of my body has spiced up our already good sex life.

A twenty-eight-year-old man wrote:

After some coaxing and seeing it done in a XXX video my current girlfriend has started to pay attention to my nipples. At first it didn't do that much for me, but we have found that it takes much more pressure for a man to feel what a woman feels. She started by tweaking me occasionally, and as time has passed I have become much more sensitive and much more responsive. She can easily make me hard by pinching and pulling my nipples, and it felt incredible the few times her pinches coincided with my orgasm. I would advise others to give it a try. Patience and persistence will pay off.

A forty-year-old man wrote:

My nipples are now very sensitive but it took some training from an attentive and very erotic woman. She spent time on them. She licked them, tweaked them, and, as I approached orgasm, twisted them. Now if she comes up behind me, slides her hands down my chest, and rubs my nipples, they stand at attention . . . as does another part of my body.

Okay, you get the idea. Of course, we know that women really enjoy breast play.

How to Give It for Him

A few notes on playing with a woman's breasts:

- Be gentle. Caress, don't press.

- If you want to squeeze, do it gently. Use your whole hand, not just your fingers.

- Don't just aim for the nipple; stroke all parts of a woman's breast.

- Use swirling motions, avoiding the areola and nipple area, teasing by getting closer and closer to the center without actually touching it.

- Use oil or lotion if you like to increase the sensation. Get even kinkier by using a small piece of sandpaper, lightly scratched over her nipple.

- If you want to play with temperature, use a warm cloth or an ice cube on her skin.

- Eventually, when her nipple is erect, play with it. Pull lightly, and pinch. Twist, keeping it very gentle until she lets you know that she wants more. And she will.

- Use your mouth. Kiss your way to the center, then lick and suck. Let her reactions guide you as to exactly how hard.

- Small bites inflame. Again, use her moans and body language tell you how much pressure to use.

- Take your time.

- Take your time.

- Take your time.

A *twenty-eight-year-old woman* wrote:
I love having my breasts played with. Oh God, sometimes, if it's done right, I love it more than sexual intercourse itself.

Start out rubbing them, just to get them congested and heated up. Mine actually get bigger when I'm excited that way. Then I like for him to run his fingers repeatedly over my nipples and areola till they get hard and puffy.

I like oral sensations a lot. I like my guy to squeeze my tits while licking them furiously with his tongue, but most importantly he has to suck on them! I always get the best feeling when he doesn't just suck the nipple itself, but tugs a good portion of my breast flesh into his mouth. I go soooo crazy once a guy starts sucking on my breasts that I'll usually let a guy suck on them as long as he wants to. I like it when his hands are doing other things too.

Breast play is one of God's most gracious gifts to us women.

A *fifty-year-old man* wrote:
My wife has small breasts with large, sensitive nipples, and she frequently needs to have her nipples

sucked, rubbed, or played with in order to climax. Once I start to stimulate her breasts, however, she comes very quickly, so I have to hold off until she's had time to build up to a satisfying climax.

Once she's ready for it, she loves to have her nipples sucked, or one sucked and the other rubbed, or sometimes both played with. It depends. Breast play is an important part of sex with us.

It wasn't always this way. We've been together twelve years, but only in the last four or five have her breasts become so sensitive. Before that she enjoyed breast play only moderately. I was the one who loved to have my nipples stimulated and I still do. Rubbing my nipples makes me very hard, and if I'm already hard, it makes me come almost immediately. My wife has used this to devastating effect on many occasions.

A *thirty-one-year-old woman* wrote:

I love having my breasts played with and the longer the better. Although my breasts are small my nipples are quite large and very sensitive. Playing with them right can bring me to orgasm all by itself. I love to have them sucked, squeezed, and yes even the nipples bitten gently (or not so gently) but not so hard that it causes more pain than pleasure. I want to feel that the man is there, not just see him.

A *twenty-eight-year-old woman* wrote:

I love to have my breasts fondled. In fact, having my breasts fondled causes my orgasms to be more intense. I like my partner to start out very slowly and gently and roll my nipples between his fingers. Like most other women, I just love for them to be sucked on, even when I go to sleep. It's very important for me that my partner knows how to touch my breasts.

How to Get It for Her

Encourage your partner to play with your breasts and nipples. Moan, squirm, and don't hesitate to use your hands to show him just how and where you want to be squeezed. Of course, if you can, tell your partner just how good it feels and what gets you hottest. Better still, show him by letting him watch as you play with your breasts and nipples. Suggest that he put his hands on yours while you stroke, pinch, pull, et cetera.

Lots of women wrote and said that they can climax from breast stimulation alone.

A forty-three-year-old woman wrote:
I don't think I'm the only woman who can come from having a guy play with my nipples, both with his fingers and his mouth. God, just sucking can do it for me. It's difficult to convince a man that it's that good, but I think my reactions (I moan, scream, and almost cry from the excitement) eventually show him. It's amazing for us both.

A fifty-one-year-old man wrote:
I don't know whether it was this lady's perfect orgasm but it sure looked great from out here. She totally amazed me by being able to come from

breast stimulation alone. We got a little drunk one evening during a business weekend seminar and went back to my room. She was wearing a really soft blue sweater (I can picture it now although it was almost fifteen years ago) and I began to stroke her through it.

Eventually I pulled it off and unsnapped her bra. I still remember being amazed that I could still do that with one hand. Anyway, I began to roll her large nipples between my thumb and first finger and it seemed to drive her crazy. I kneaded and sucked and generally enjoyed myself as she got higher and higher. Well, suddenly her back arched and she grabbed my hand and held it against her tit.

She told me later that she had climaxed and, from her wetness when I entered her a few minutes later I don't doubt it.

Erotic Massage

Let your fingers do the walking? Absolutely. There's a lot to be learned about your partner's body, and much of it can be done with a full-body massage. Where is he most sensitive? What parts of her body make her squirm?

Body mapping is a deliberate attempt to discover your partner's erogenous zones. You all know that guys like their penis and testicles stroked, and a woman goes for breasts and genitals. But there are lots of other places that can curl your partner's toes. Try the following:

- The inside of your partner's elbows and the backs of knees.

- Your partner's sides and belly.

- The back of the neck.

- Underarms.

- Feet and toes.

- Fingers and between them.

Use your palms, your fingertips, your nails (lightly). Use light, gentle touches and firm strokes. Any and all of those spots might be the "magic button" you've been searching for. One quick note: Many of my writers agree that a woman wants her massage to last longer than a man does. Guide yourself accordingly. Encourage your partner to tell you when it's not pleasurable anymore. If he's falling asleep rather than reveling in the sensual pleasure, it's time to move on. On this note, she might want to explore one area each lovemaking session, then go for the gold.

How to Give It

- Make sure your hands are smooth and soft. Use hand lotion on them first if you need to, and trim your fingernails so there are no sharp edges.

- Turn up the heat in the house.

- To protect the bedding, spread a plastic sheet— you can get them at the hardware store for painting— or use an old plastic tablecloth or shower curtain over the bed and cover that with a soft, thick towel.

- At the beginning, cover his or her body with another

towel and expose only the part you're working on.

- Use a light massage oil. Specialty products are available through Web sites and catalogs, but baby oil or plain vegetable oil work fine. If you're going to spend a lot of time, baby or mineral oil tends to thicken, so try avocado or jojoba oil. If you're in doubt, rub a little between your fingers and see how it feels.

- Don't keep a bottle of oil in the refrigerator for too long. It will eventually turn rancid. Just throw the old stuff out and get new.

- Warm the oil between your hands, or keep a small bottle in a bowl of warm water or a baby bottle warmer beside the bed.

- Work from the spine outward, away from the center of the body.

- Don't overlook the buttocks. Squeeze each cheek gently, pulling them apart slightly.

- Try a foot massage, playing special attention to each toe and the areas between. Treat each as if it were a penis, swirling your fingertips around it, then pulling gently. Press into the arch of the foot, then grab the heel and swivel the rest of the foot at the ankle.

- Hand massages are delicious too. Use your thumb in the palm, then rub each finger. Hold the wrist and move each hand with a gentle circular motion, as if you're turning a crank. If you're feeling adventurous, suck on each finger.

- Take your time and enjoy the sensations yourself.

Remember, you're also stroking your hands with his or her body parts.

- Enjoy.

- Enjoy.

- Enjoy.

How to Get It

A twenty-seven-year-old woman wrote:

God, I love it when my husband gives me a body rub. It all started with my bad back. It had been hurting for several weeks when a friend suggested that a back rub might relax the muscles. I asked my husband to do it for me. We got some massage oil at a store in town and, at the suggestion of the woman who sold it to us, kept it warm on a heating pad. Then I stripped to the waist, stretched out on a big towel we'd put on the bed, and he went at it. He didn't really know what he was doing but he just rubbed.

I told him just where it felt good and he really did a good job. As I relaxed, I got horny. His wonderful hands on me and all, well I wanted a "more extensive" rub. I didn't know how to ask for it so at one point I said, "Don't get fresh now." I think that gave him the idea.

Slowly his hands slipped to the sides of my breasts. I moaned and in every way I could let him know that I loved what he was doing. Well, one thing led to another and eventually he flipped me over and began to massage my front. The sex was fabulous.

My back eventually got better, but I still love my back (and front) rubs.

Oh, I've asked him whether he'd like a back rub but he always wants to just "go for the gold" so I begin with his crotch (wink, wink).

If you've always wanted any of the things in this section, ask. Remember that your partner isn't a mind reader and might not take hints. Giving him a back rub isn't a guarantee that he'll return the favor. "Love, I'd really enjoy a massage tonight. How about we meet in the bedroom in fifteen minutes? You bring the oil, I'll bring the towels." You might add, "Oh, and you bring the wine."

Chapter 4

MASTURBATION

MASTURBATION—SOMETHING MEN START AT AN early age and many women never do. I feel sorry for the woman who's never touched herself because it's really the best and most reliable way to learn about her body and what makes it sing.

Men begin to touch themselves when they begin to be potty trained and continue to be totally comfortable with their genitals. At some point they discover that it feels especially good to rub and stroke and caress; eventually they reach the age when they climax and ejaculate. Since it's embarrassing to the adults around, society tells the poor young men terrible stories about the consequences of masturbation. Most boys don't stop, they just spend tremendous amounts of time worrying about whether hair will grow on their palms, their penis will shrink, or they won't ever be able to get any pleasure out of sexual intercourse. None of those is true, by the way. Unless you really abuse your penis, masturbation does no harm.

One word about masturbation and its effects on intercourse. Over the years many men have trained their bodies to ejaculate quickly to avoid being caught doing "naughty things." This is sad because it can make a man more prone to premature ejaculation. I'll give you some hints about dealing with premature ejaculation in chapter 13.

For us women the taboos around masturbation are even stronger. We are told that it's dirty and evil—and since we really never have to touch outside the quick swipe of a sponge in the shower, we don't learn until much later, if at all, how our bodies react to various types of touch. Masturbation is really the best way to learn about your body and its orgasmic triggers.

How to Get It for Her

Ladies, I hope you've gotten past the taboo and you can freely touch where it feels good. I hope you've learned that it's your body and nothing disastrous will happen if you do things that feel nice, and that's all that masturbation is. If you haven't, the problem is where to start.

Relax. That's the first and most important thing, and maybe the most difficult. You need to get past everything you've ever learned or thought. Sensuality is beautiful, and you're entitled to it. Period.

Find a comfortable and private place to experiment. It might be in bed in the dark or in the shower or bath. Wherever you choose, you need space, time, and most of all lots and lots of privacy. Orgasm isn't going to happen in a few moments or even in a few masturbating sessions. It takes time and patience. And it certainly isn't going to happen if you have one ear on the front door, waiting for the kids to get home from school.

For me, it took several evenings in the bathtub, touching where it felt good and satisfying my curiosity about my body. For any of you who feel that you're beyond this, I was thirty at the time and had two school-age children. I touched, explored, and felt incredibly guilty for a while. It took months before I tried sliding a toothbrush handle into my vagina and still longer before I inserted my fingers for pleasure.

I can't say it often enough. It's your body and you're allowed—no, encouraged—to touch it.

Once you've found the place and time, find out what will help get you excited. For me, it was erotic literature, romance novels with great sex scenes. For you, it might be music or an erotic film. Maybe there's a scene in an R- or even PG-rated movie that curls your toes. Whatever it is, use it as kindling and stoke the flames with whatever you can. Alcohol? Sure, why not. A glass of wine or beer will certainly relax you.

Then touch. Think about what turns you on during lovemaking. Your nipples? The insides of your thighs? Breast play? Soft caresses or scratches with fingernails? Eventually your fingers will migrate to your vagina. Explore. By now you should be wet, so feel that. Slippery? Copious fluids or just a bit? If you're not wet, be patient. It might not happen this session or even the next. This is new territory, new sensations, and there are a lot of taboos to get past.

Can you find your clitoris? That's the nub of tissue between the fleshy, hairy lips. You'll find it if you part those lips and slide your fingers down through your pubic hair and then between them. You won't have to go far. How will it feel? The clitoris is made of erectile tissue. This means that, like a penis, as you get more aroused the tissue gets larger and harder. So in the beginning your clitoris can be difficult to find, but as your excitement grows, so does your clit, making it easier and easier to locate. You'll have a pretty good gauge of how excited you are by how prominent your clitoris becomes.

Find the places that feel the best and stroke there. Do you like to touch the top of your clit or just the sides? Left side or right, or do both feel the same? As you get more excited, change the touches. Maybe early on you like them firm, but later softer ones feel better. Do you want to put your fingers inside? If you do, do it. Thrust? Slide? Not at all? Whatever!

Eventually, as you masturbate, you'll find that the touches

will become more urgent, and eventually you'll climax. Amazingly enough, you might not even recognize it when it happens. You might not have violent spasms or shaking or any of the other body movements you've been led to expect from popular romance novels. You will, however, notice a lessening of tension. Great. When it no longer feels good to stroke, stop. Then do it again next time.

By masturbating, you're also training your body to respond to those touches, teaching it the path to orgasm, and eventually to the perfect orgasm. As you learn, you'll be better able to teach your partner. Touch here. Softly. Touch there. Hard.

Once you learn to masturbate, you can do it during sex, while he watches, or instead of intercourse when he's not available.

Lots of women masturbate, and they have different techniques.

A thirty-two-year-old woman wrote:

I masturbate often, even though I've been married for four years. My husband travels and while he's away I get so horny that I just have to do something. I've printed out lots of stories from various sites on the Net and when I get too hungry to wait I stretch out on the bed, take off my jeans, and read a few. When I'm ready to explode from the excitement, I get out my vibrator and touch myself in just the right places then boom. It just happens.

I used to stop there, but recently I've been able to get aroused again and come two or even three times. I would recommend it for any woman.

A twenty-six-year-old woman wrote:

I've been masturbating since I was in my teens. The first time I was reading a sexy book and felt all itchy between my legs. It was really difficult for me to touch, since I'd been told not to and had my hand slapped a few times by my mother when I was a kid. Anyway, I did and, well you can imagine my surprise when I came. I wasn't even sure what it was but I knew it felt really good.

Over the years I've perfected my technique. I've even shown my husband how I like to be touched and he's watched me do it. It makes me so hot when he says, "Show me how you masturbate when I'm not around." And I do. It's great.

A twenty-seven-year-old woman wrote:

I love to surf the Web, looking for pictures of hunky guys pleasuring themselves. When I find one I particularly like I pretend that he's in the room with me, touching himself and watching me do the same. My fingers play between my legs and eventually I get out my big dildo, close my eyes, and pretend that he's fucking me. It feels great and makes me much calmer and better able to deal with my very complicated life. Am I justifying it? Maybe, but I think I still have a few of those early lectures by my mother in my brain.

How to Get It for Him

I thought I'd let some of the men who've written to me tell you how they masturbate. I would assume that most of you guys do it from time to time, but maybe you can still learn a trick or two.

A thirty-two-year-old man wrote:

Recently I did something different! I undressed

and shaved all my pubic hair off until I was as smooth and clean as a ten-year-old boy. I then set up my video camera focused on my genital area and began filming myself masturbating. I rubbed my penis slowly and then fast until I was stiff and swollen, then I let my penis slowly go limp again before playing with it again until I had a full erection.

When playing the tape back, I got to see a different view of my penis as it was played with. I could see my balls turning and bouncing inside my scrotum as I stroked, and I slowed the tape down when I ejaculated. It's a turn-on to see the semen stream and shoot from my penis in slow motion. I also played the tape for my girlfriend, and she masturbated to orgasm watching my solo sex movie.

A fifty-year-old man wrote:

I have discovered that long periods of self-stimulation are so gratifying that I would almost rather masturbate than have sex with my girlfriend. When you play with yourself, you don't have to worry about time limits, or anything else that might make the mood wrong with a partner. I love to have masturbation sessions that last two or more hours, and the final release is beyond description.

I begin by undressing and sitting nude at my computer while visiting sites that have erotic material. I have found new areas of pleasure on and around my genitals to touch as I read and look at things that arouse me. I gently rub my testicles, the area between my anus and scrotum, pull on the head of my penis, and play with my shaft. I've also discovered that I like to play with my nipples.

My erections are hard, and the pre-ejaculate flows out and forms a small pool on the floor as I stimulate myself. Sometimes I reach a point that when I touch any part of my genitals I can't help but moan out from the incredible soothing feeling of the level of pleasure I can achieve.

Right before ejaculation, my penis is so stiff that I feel like any further blood flow will cause it to explode. I watch the head swell and turn a shade of purple at the glans, and I stroke the shaft slowly until a small amount of semen flows out of the head of my penis. Then there's an explosion as the fluid shoots up several inches. My legs are shaking, I'm moaning out and grasping my penis shaft and scrotum in spastic response to a wonderful orgasm.

These orgasms are the most powerful I have ever felt, and nobody can say that self-stimulation is second best to real sex with a partner because it depends on how you approach it. Perfect orgasms? Maybe, and I'm still trying to make them better.

A forty-five-year-old man wrote:
I have found that it is very stimulating to play with myself while looking into a mirror. I like to take a shower and then stand nude in front of the full-length one on the back of the bathroom door. I then look over my naked body as the excitement level rises and I can watch my hands and my penis as I pleasure myself. If you've never watched yourself, you should give it a try.

Mutual Masturbation

Watching your lover masturbate and masturbating together are wonderful ways to learn about what creates the maximum heat.

How to Get It

Encourage your partner to touch him- or herself during lovemaking. "I love to watch your hands on your body." As one writer suggested, "Show me how you pleasure yourself when I'm not around." It might take a while to convince your partner that it's really okay, but when you do, the fun begins.

Another approach might be to get your partner really aroused, then stop all activities. Place his or her hand in the right spot and say that you won't do anything more until you've gotten some guidance. Then turn up your antennae and learn. You can also place your hand over your partner's and use it to stroke all the places you know arouse.

At first it will probably be really embarrassing, but it's a delicious embarrassment. With some encouragement, though, it will happen and you'll both get a lot of pleasure and education from it.

A twenty-seven-year-old man wrote:

> My girl and I had been dating for a while when she
> suggested we masturbate for each other. I watched
> as she rubbed just above her clitoral hood, and I
> suddenly realized that I had been touching her
> vulva all wrong during sex play. I always tried to
> expose her clitoris, and she always pulled back
> because it was too sensitive for her. It was quite a
> revelation for me and I've been touching her more
> gently since. Maybe that was what she was trying
> to show me.

After she came, I played with myself in front of her and masturbated the way I do when I'm alone. I pulled on the glans of my penis while gently rubbing my testicles, and she too discovered that her way of touching me was a little off.

During foreplay now, I rub her genitals the way I saw her touch herself, and I can bring her to orgasm this way. It also feels so good to have her touching my penis and scrotum the way I do, and when I come from her touching me this way I yell loudly because it feels so good.

Everyone should masturbate in front of their significant other. You'll be amazed at what you can learn about creating a better orgasm.

A twenty-six-year-old woman wrote:
On the subject of masturbation, I'm in a four-year relationship with a forty-year-old man. He is so sexy to me and has such an incredibly beautiful cock . . . not because it's big, but because it's so proportionately perfect. Nothing excites me more than to see him caressing and manipulating his own sweet package. I love the way he grabs his balls occasionally while stroking the shaft and head.

Watching him gives me great insight into the sensitive areas on his body and how I can actually touch his balls! I was always afraid I'd hurt him by touching him there. I've been a cock worshiper and lover of oral sex all my sexually active life, but I have always been kind of afraid to be too rough with a man's sac. I've seen how just a simple bump in the wrong spot can render a man helpless. I remember all those times the boys in school would drop to their knees in pain from getting hit with a ball or something. Well, I was really afraid of turning a sensual situation into unwanted horrific pain. Until I saw a man handling himself, I really had no idea what or where was okay.

Now I do things that give pleasure that I would have shied away from before. Boy, what we had been missing! Men should realize the best way to teach a lover is to show her!

A thirty-eight-year-old woman wrote:

I love to watch a man perform self-pleasure—it makes me so wet. I'm not sure why I find it so exciting, maybe because self-pleasure is viewed as taboo.

When I ask my current lover to masturbate, I cuddle close to him, nibble on his neck and ears, and whisper fantasies to him to heighten his arousal. I love to watch his cock get so hard as his hand strokes. By watching him pleasure himself, I have learned how to stroke his dick with my hands and I know what areas of his cock are sensitive and tease it with my tongue and mouth.

Masturbation can become a delicious part of your lovemaking, and touching yourself and your partner can be a tremendous turn-on.

A fifty-year-old man wrote:

My wife and I have been happily married for thirty-one years. Let me tell you a bit about our sex life.

When we were newlyweds, we had hot, steamy animal sex—constantly fucking and sucking—but we didn't broach the subject of masturbation. She must have suspected I jerked off; there was always a well-thumbed men's magazine lying around, but she never talked about it.

One night we got pretty drunk and I made a comment about jacking off on her. She said, "Go ahead!" I agreed to, but only if after I did it, she would show me how she touched herself. It was a done deal.

My heart raced as I pulled down my jeans and briefs and began stroking my already semi-hard erection to its full size. As I caressed myself, I shifted my gaze between my cock and her face. Somehow her watching me made it all the more exciting, and I was unable to take the "long road home." I came almost immediately.

She was very aroused by my display of self-pleasure. "Okay, your turn," I said. She shyly pulled down her jeans and panties, soaked with pussy juice, and began a rapid back and forth rubbing on her clit and lips. It didn't take her long either to reach a screaming climax; her body first became rigid with ecstasy, then she collapsed in a heap.

Ever since that night's display, masturbation has been an integral part of our sexual activities. We have sex at least one night a week and share masturbation of one another. We masturbate privately as well and enjoy telling each other hot tidbits of our solo playtime. We have our own toy boxes, each filled with a variety of delights; she has several dildos, including her favorite pink jelly cock that is normal size. She also has a long black one with a handle, which she uses when she really wants to show off for me.

My toy box has some jelly sleeve masturbators: a newer tighter one and a more broken in looser one. I also enjoy some smaller butt plugs and slender anal vibrators occasionally.

Recently we've begun taking pictures of each other masturbating, both on stills and video. It's so much better than looking at a magazine or pictures on the Web. I watch and tell myself, "That's my wife doing that deliciously naughty stuff."

A *twenty-seven-year-old woman* wrote:

My boyfriend and I like to watch each other while we masturbate, but we have never watched when the other didn't know it. Then my boyfriend came up with the hottest idea! He told me that he sometimes sits at the computer and plays with himself while looking at sex pictures of nude women. He said that since he gets home about two hours before I do, that's when he masturbates the most. He suggested that I could come home one night, walk around to the side of the house where the computer room is, and look through the spaces in the blinds to see if he was playing with himself. He said this way he would be turned on thinking I might be watching, and I would be turned on by catching him without him really knowing. So each night on my way home I would be a little excited because of the prospect of catching him masturbating.

Two weeks went by, and I hadn't caught him. I only saw him at the computer, but not much else. Then on a Friday I came home, walked to the window, and peeked in. There he was sitting with just a T-shirt on, nude from the waist down. My heart rate jumped, and a wave of excitement came over me as I anticipated the show. For ten minutes he sat there looking and surfing on the computer, but no masturbation yet.

Then he must have seen something good on the screen because I saw his penis swell. He began to rub his scrotum and testicles and his stiff penis moved back and forth as the stimulation continued. He touched his penis head with his fingertips then switched back to rubbing his balls. I looked around to see if anyone was watching me peep through the window. My boyfriend then wiped some pre cum off the tip of his penis and tasted it. I was getting so hot that I thought I'd come right then.

I could not help it anymore. I unzipped my jeans a little, slipped my hand beneath my panties, and began to rub the hood of my clitoris with the lubrication that was flowing freely out of my vagina. A few minutes later my boyfriend removed his shirt and was fully naked as he then began to stroke his erect penis faster and faster. This was a treat because I have never seen this type of masturbation. He was rubbing his scrotum and stroking his penis until jism came shooting up and out of his stiff cock.

It was then that I had a wonderful orgasm too. I zipped up and went into the house. My boyfriend looked a little surprised but said he hoped that this was the time I was watching. Just talking about it made us both hot again and we made love on the kitchen floor.

What a wonderful sexy experience watching someone masturbate when they are unaware.

Masturbating while your partner watches can be a wonderful teaching tool for both of you. You can each improve your orgasm and your partner's by showing and learning what you each like. And don't overlook masturbation as a way to get your heat rising as part of foreplay. You can stop short of climax, then get together for intercourse.

Chapter 5

INTERCOURSE

THE JOURNEY'S DESTINATION, THE ULTIMATE filling for our sexual sandwich, is intercourse. Before we begin, here's a letter that emphasizes the importance of communication, the key to achieving the perfect orgasm.

A forty-year-old woman wrote:

I used to be afraid of trying to give my husband a hand job because I thought there were things I didn't know how to do and I was afraid both of embarrassing myself and failing my husband. How silly I was.

One evening he asked me why I never touched him and, after lots of hemming and hawing, I told him. He laughed, not *at* me but *with* me. Then he took my hand and used it to stroke his cock. He patiently showed me just where he liked to be touched, how hard and how fast. It took several nights before I felt brave enough to initiate it, but now I feel like an expert and I love what it does to and for him.

Soon I'm going to suggest that I teach him exactly how I like to be touched.

Positions and Such

I get dozens of letters asking, "Can you suggest some new positions?" My answer is always the same: Sexual positions flow from one to another. Everyone has different preferences—what might work for me or another couple might not be your cup of tea. My best advice is to try everything and see what works for you. During a lovemaking session, Ed and I might be in half a dozen different positions or more.

Here's a great idea: Try them all. Let's hear it for experimentation.

I recently surveyed visitors to my Web site about their favorite positions. You can read all the wonderful things they had to say in my book *Naughty Secrets*. The following are a few of their favorites:

- Man on top.

- Woman on top.

- Doggy-style with him entering her from behind while she's on all fours.

- Scissors, where they lie in an X shape with legs intertwined.

- Side by side.

- Curled, spoon-style.

- Standing, including against a wall.

- Standing doggy-style with her bent over and him grasping her hips from behind.

Don't forget the furniture:

- In a chair.

- On a lounger, which can really heat things up if you take a moment to consider.

- With her partly on and partly off the dining room table or sitting on the kitchen counter.

The first three positions seemed to be the most common, but all the ones listed here were mentioned. If you're really interested in changing your normal position, read on.

Man on top, the traditional missionary position, has the advantage of being the most familiar and most comfortable, but for the woman it's the one least likely to provide clitoral stimulation, something most women need to achieve orgasm. Man on top is the best for a woman who's attempting to get pregnant. It also leaves her hands free to play with his body. Many men have sensitive nipples, so she might pinch or scratch to see whether it gets the desired reaction. She can also reach around and cup or stroke his testicles or the particularly sensitive area between the testicles and anus. It's a long reach, but with a bit of wiggling it can be done—and it's worth it.

The woman-on-top positions, both prone and straddling, need the firmest penis and therefore might not be the best for men who are having difficulty achieving or maintaining an erection, or those who have problems getting from semi-erect to erect. Using this position also provides the least chance for her to get pregnant, but don't count on this for any kind of birth control. Women, when you're on top you can move as you like, varying the depth and angle of his penetration. He can play with your breasts and rub your clitoris, so encourage him to. If he's not immediately interested, show him what you like.

Both these front-to-front positions give both partners access to their lover's body, for hands and mouths to roam. During intercourse, don't neglect your partner's body. Your hands should never be still.

Which position is best for you? It depends on what you want. Face-to-face positions allow you to look at each other and touch, caress, and play with your partner. Standing can be particularly arousing, but you may want to be horizontal in case your knees give out. You don't want to have to depend on your guy to hold you up. Man behind allows him to reach around and play with his partner's breasts and stroke her clitoris, but it denies her the ability to easily touch him. This can be particularly arousing if done facing a mirror so you can both see what's happening. The combination of participating and watching is delicious.

Simultaneous Orgasm

A word about simultaneous orgasms. Couples have written to me asking whether there were special techniques to achieve simultaneous orgasm, the supposed best way to climax. In my opinion, simultaneous orgasms aren't very important. If you two happen to come at the same time, great. If not, let orgasm happen when it happens. Just make sure neither partner is left unsatisfied.

Ed and I have tried for simultaneous orgasm, but it seems to me that one of us is rushing while the other is waiting. On the other hand, once I've climaxed I can enjoy Ed's path to the perfect orgasm and help him along. He does the same for me. That's a pleasure I would miss if we always came together.

Multiple Orgasms

On the topic of multiple orgasms, here's an interesting and quite valuable way of looking at it. If your version of an orgasm is one that leaves you satisfied, then one may be enough. However, if you look at an orgasm as a peak of pleasure that can lead to another, that's fine too. I guess it's the difference between a gigantic pastrami sandwich with Russian dressing and coleslaw with a side order of french fries and a chocolate shake, after which you can't eat another bite, versus tiny little open-face sandwiches that you nibble throughout the day.

If snacking is what you're aiming for, fine. The best way to do that would be to hold something back from your first climax so you have something left for the next, and the next.

A forty-one-year-old woman wrote:

> The first time I came more than once was quite a revelation. I never knew that my body was capable of something like that. It happened with my husband after three years of marriage. We'd made love and both of us had come. For the first time, he continued to stroke my clit, very lightly, while we caught our breath. I found that I was getting hot again and really didn't know whether my body was capable of another orgasm, but my hunger just kept growing. I put my hand over his and showed him where I wanted him to touch me, and after just a few minutes I came again. It wasn't as violent as the previous one, but it was fabulous. He was as surprised and delighted as I was.
>
> From then on he's been a darling and makes sure I don't want another climax when we've both come. Sometimes I do, sometimes I don't. It's all terrific.

Most of those who can achieve multiple orgasms are women, but I'm assured that men can too. They can train their bodies to hold back until they can delay orgasm indefinitely and allow it to happen when they want and as often as they want.

A forty-year-old man wrote:

Women are capable of multiple orgasms during foreplay and intercourse; however, if a man has an orgasm during foreplay, he usually loses his erection, sexual desire, and can't fulfill his partner's desire for sexual intercourse. My wife and I discovered that it doesn't have to be that way.

After sharing sex together for several years, we made an accidental discovery. One afternoon, I was aroused and approached her. We closed the curtains, folded down the bedcovers, and enjoyed a long session of foreplay. Just prior to intercourse, I lay on my back while she lubricated my penis for the ensuing penetration.

Taking a tube of K-Y Jelly from the nightstand, she squeezed some onto her hand and then spread it on my penis. Next, using a plastic squeeze bottle, she squirted a tiny stream of water on my penis. The water mixed with the K-Y Jelly and my cock really got slippery. She spread this slick mess around my penis by sliding her hand up the shaft and over the head of my cock, and then back down again. My cock, still extremely sensitive from our foreplay, nearly exploded. "Oh God stop!" I said as my cock jerked to her touch.

"Want me to bring it off?" she asked, still holding my cock.

I wanted to come right then and there but I said, "Let it go," hoping it wasn't too late. As we watched my cock, a small blob of milky white come slowly oozed out and the jerking stopped. My orgasm subsided as the come released.

Thinking it was too late, I relaxed, feeling fulfilled. Except for the flow of the milky white come, this incident was a not-unusual foreplay occurrence. I love being brought close to orgasm then coming back down. On this afternoon my wife straddled me and pushed my still erect cock into her pussy. It stayed hard as she squirmed around getting comfy. I told her that I just had my orgasm and would probably get soft.

She began fucking me, her cunt gliding up and down my superslick cock. To our amazement, we enjoyed over ten minutes of continuous coitus, ending when I had another orgasm inside her. This second orgasm was just like it had always been. My ejaculate released in searing spurts, my erection softened, and we were done.

Since then we've pushed this process until I can come—or get close—then allow my erection to subside. Sometimes I ejaculate a small amount at the peak of pleasure, then can ejaculate again, and again. Can anyone do this? I think so, and it's really fabulous.

Spontaneity Versus Planning

Many books on sexuality tout spontaneity as the best path to the perfect orgasm, and if you can be spontaneous, that's wonderful.

Grab her, throw her onto the sofa, and have your way with her. Drag him into the bedroom, pull off his belt, and go for it. Delightful. This can be a wonderful part of vacation, for example. You're lounging on the beach and things start to heat up. You look at your partner and together you grab your towels and dash for the bed. Bravo!

One hot Sunday afternoon or a really cold Tuesday evening you just give each other that signal and go for it. Have you ever done it in front of the Christmas tree when the kids are sleeping soundly?

How many of us can do that, however? Very few. We don't have the time or space to "just do it." So we plan. And what's wrong with that? Remember back when you two were dating? You had a date on Saturday night and you knew you'd end up in bed. Did that spoil your pleasure? I think not. Actually it probably made you hot all day, just thinking about what was up and coming.

Stop expecting things that you're told should be good. Make the most of what you've got. Set the mood for the evening. Plan what underwear you're going to wear. Don't eat garlic for dinner unless your partner indulges too. Buy scented candles and/or flowers for the bedroom. Rent a sexy video and tell your partner that you'll watch it together, later. Plan an hour together to surf the Net for sexy letters or adult Web sites. Or pull out this book and read some of the letters together or bookmark some pages to read early in the day, then anticipate what the evening will bring. Indulge.

Places

If you've always made love in the bedroom, you've missed a lot. Your house is filled with rooms, and you haven't really lived until you've made love in every one. Try the dining room table, the coffee table, or the kitchen counter—which, by the way is at a perfect height for oral sex. I knew a couple once who broke three toilet seats within the first few years of their marriage. Hmmm.

If you want to be romantic and make love in front of a fire, be sure to use a soft towel beneath your behind. Rug burns are a pain in the behind—literally—been there, done that.

Be adventurous. Make love in the shower or in a hot tub or pool, in the backyard, or on the kids' swing set. If you do it in the lounge chair, you'll never look at it the same way again. How about doing it the park at 2 A.M.? When I was dating, cars had bench seats in the front, which made lovemaking in the front seat possible. Now, thanks to bucket seats and center consoles, it's difficult to make love without moving to the backseat. So do that. Doing it on the washing machine during the spin cycle has become a bit of a joke—but why not? The ultimate vibrator for both of you?

Be creative and climb out of your rut.

Times

Again, shake it up. If you always make love in the evening, wake your partner up with a suggestion, or just jump his or her bones. Make love in the afternoon sometime. You can add to the excitement by opening a sunny window and letting the heat shine on your partner's genitals—if you have no nosy neighbors, of course.

The G-Spot

I think, by now, it's pretty well proven that there is such a thing as a g-spot. This pad of tissue, named for Ernest Grafenberg, wraps around the urethra and, when massaged, seems to give some women extra sexual pleasure.

How to Give It for Him

A woman's g-spot is found on the belly side of her vaginal channel about a finger's length from the opening. The best way to reach it is to insert one finger, curved toward her belly button, and try to find a thickened section of tissue deep inside. Then experiment by stroking and pressing. Ask her to tell you whether this feels good. If it does, do more. If she says she doesn't notice any difference, and you've "looked around" as much as you can, forget about it.

A thirty-one-year-old woman wrote:

> I am very orgasmic and achieve many climaxes easily by myself or with my partner. I learned how to pleasure myself with clitoral stimulation at a young age, but my most memorable orgasm came the first time a man stimulated my g-spot. Maybe it was the novelty of the experience, but with the memory still burning ten years later I think it approached perfection.
>
> I was in my first year of college, and, after a brief flirtation, found myself sharing a bed with an upperclassman. Reluctant to surrender my virginity, but sexually curious, I allowed him to slip his hand inside my underwear. With magnet-like instincts, he found my g-spot and began caressing it, slowly at first, but soon gaining intensity. I felt waves traveling throughout my body, and he increased his speed in response to my cries and moans. The pleasure seemed to multiply and soon became so overwhelming that my legs felt numb and I nearly lost all feeling in them.

I grabbed the bed's headboard and continued to moan and pant as the pleasure went on relentlessly. After more than an hour, the stimulation ceased and I was completely exhausted, but the warm sensation in my g-spot remained and my legs were a bit weak. Unfortunately, things didn't work out between us and this was the only encounter we had. Boy, am I grateful for that one night with a guy with such skillful hands!

Hand Jobs

If you always play the same way and end with intercourse, you might be missing something special. Have you ever used your hands to actually bring your partner to climax? Maybe you did when you two were dating and you didn't have any other way to scratch that sexual itch. I fondly remember the front seat of my then-boyfriend's Ford. We could each climax without actual intercourse. Phew—delicious.

How to Give It for Her

Giving a genital massage to a guy is something women have to learn and practice, practice, practice.

- If you're going to do a lot of rubbing, use a lubricant. Slippery feels wonderful.

- Touch lightly, then more firmly. Stroke from base to tip, then tip to base, and see which he likes best. He'll probably like both.

- Wrap your fingers around the shaft and, while squeezing lightly, stroke the head with the palm or fingertips of the other hand.

- Twist lightly, either quickly or slowly. Change pace occasionally and see what makes him groan.

- Stroke one hand from tip to base and, before it reaches bottom, start the same stroke again with the other hand.

- Place your palms against his shaft, then ask him to cover your hands with his. Let him show you what strokes he likes—a great way to learn.

- Learn to enjoy it for yourself. Remember you're also stroking your palms with his penis.

I asked my visitors about the old-fashioned hand job.

A fifty-one-year-old man wrote:

My wife has been jacking me off since before we were married. We have been married twenty-six years and I still enjoy it very much. My wife loves being in control and teasing my cock. She jacks me off in several positions with many different strokes.

She uses several techniques to get me even more excited. I love her breasts so when she removes her bra and her tits spill out it drives me crazy. She slows up a little so I can play with her tits but it isn't long before my cock explodes.

She also enjoys stripping for me and playing with her own tits while I jack myself off. I must admit it is kind of erotic for me to jack off while she watches.

A fifty-seven-year-old man wrote:

I love a good hand job. My wife will do me whenever I want her to. When we shower together, she will always soap me up and get me off. She will also give me a hand job in bed or put on a show for me using one of her vibrators while I jack off watching her getting off. My wife is an expert at giving hand jobs and yes, she is good at other sex acts as well. The good old hand job is alive and well at our house!

A twenty-eight-year-old man wrote:

Hand jobs—I love them! They are so intimate and I can just concentrate on really enjoying it.

This is how my lady does it. It starts with the warm-up. I love the feeling of her hand rubbing my cock through my trousers until it gets hard as she kisses me. Then as things progress she unzips me and removes my trousers and boxers, exposing my now hard cock and balls. I can't wait for her to touch it. She's in control and loves it. She touches and plays with my shaft by bouncing it around a little and pulling it away from my body, enjoying its hardness.

That first touch is a great feeling and satisfies my urgent need. She takes her shirt and bra off to give me extra stimulation and looks into my eyes to see my horny reaction. She wraps her hand around my cock snugly and starts to stroke it up and down slowly. She says she likes seeing her hand wrapped around me and making me hard. I also watch her hand on me and look into her eyes to see how much she's enjoying giving me pleasure.

After some time she starts to increase the speed of her pumping until my balls are bouncing around. I'm watching her as much as I can despite my heavy breathing and the eye-closing ecstasy. She makes sure to rub that sensitive nerve area at the bottom of my cock head at the point nearest my body on every stroke. It feels soooo good.

Now she starts talking to me as she continues to pump me. "Oh, you're so hard, and so big. I'm getting so wet while I'm stroking your big hard cock." She can see and feel me getting really, really turned on, and I'm as hard as I can get.

At this point we enter a new level of talk. She can see I'm at my peak as she looks up at me. I'm breathing hard and writhing around, reveling in the feeling of her hand pumping up and down my hard cock. She usually makes sexy comments like, "God, it feels so good to see you so hot. I can't describe how good. I want you to come."

I can feel the come starting to move from my balls. I can't speak to tell her but she knows. "Come on, give me your come. I want you to spurt your hot love juice." At this point I'm a goner. A perfect orgasm almost every time.

After about a minute I can finally kiss her hard to show her how great that was. Then, when I can catch my breath, I start stroking her. She's already so wet that it's easy to make her come using only my hands.

Of course we have intercourse often, but this way of making love is very special to us.

A twenty-seven-year-old man wrote:

My wife and I give hand jobs to one another at least once a week. Sometimes it's just the right thing to do. It feels good, not superior to anything else, just pleasantly different. She uses a hand lotion on me (well named I might add) while I use my bare hand on her. Her climaxes are a sight to behold as she thrashes about and screams with delight.

I lie on my back and she leans over me and begins by spreading the lotion over by cock and balls. Sometimes the lotion is cold, but that just increases the pleasure for me. She often nudges my legs apart and plays with my anal opening with a lubed finger. She doesn't insert all the way, but rims the opening and teases me with her fingertip. She usually does me with her right hand, but switches once in a while to her weaker left. It's funny that her two hands feel so different.

It feels great when she uses her free hand to play with and massage my balls. She will stretch them out against my thigh and roll them around like a couple of hard-boiled eggs in a lubed pouch. As I approach my climax she intensifies the pulling and aims the tip like a fire hose. My legs jiggle and my body squirms until I finally let go with several blasts of come. She continues to milk me until I shrivel back to normal. We've learned to keep a towel near the bed to use as a target and to clean up afterward.

A fifty-four-year-old man wrote:

I absolutely love to be jerked off. My wife and I

have developed ways of doing it in public, in restaurants, movie theaters, et cetera. My favorite is doing it at a restaurant where they have fairly long tablecloths. She sometimes will work on my cock for twenty to thirty minutes, alternating between very delicate, very slow motions and all-out jacking. She usually brings a small travel tube of K-Y Jelly and sometimes she surprises me with it.

A forty-year-old man wrote:

My most erotic fantasy is having a woman talk to me through a hand job, trying to distract me. She would ask me questions and make me answer, make me concentrate, all the while driving me closer to the edge—toying with me, teasing me.

"Do you like strawberry pie?"

"Um . . . yeah, I guess."

"No, for real."

"Yeah."

"What other kind of pie?"

That slows everything down and sort of forces me to try to do two things at once. It's so exciting.

A sixty-one-year-old man wrote:

Ahh, hand jobs. They take me back, way back, to my youth. Some of my dates were reluctant to "go all the way," or we might not have any-place private enough to take our clothes off, so we let our fingers do the walking. I've been jerked off, and returned the favor, in the library stacks, in the lobby of the girls' dorm, on a rooftop in the Bronx, and on a late-night sub-way. The risk of getting caught just increased the excitement. Sometimes something really off-beat was just the thing.

A sixty-three-year-old man wrote:

A good hand job can be more intense for a man than intercourse. I think the reason is that he is not worrying about satisfying his lover. He just relaxes and lets it happen. Same can be said for good oral sex, which usually has hand assistance.

My wife of over forty years always works my cock with her hands almost to climax. The pleasure is ongoing. Sometimes I do not make it to her pussy in time. At other times if she does not feel like sex or is tired she will get me off by hand. I always ensure that she comes by hand and or mouth. I never tire of stroking and sucking her pussy.

Hand jobs are good, just another wonderful element of good loving.

How to Give It for Him

A woman likes a man to use his fingers to arouse her just as much as a man does. Again, techniques vary, and women like different kinds of touches at different times. Check the section on oral sex for more hints.

- Stroke slowly and use her natural lubricant. If she's not lubricated yet, be more gentle and use a commercial lube if you wish.

- Explore the folds.

- I know I've said this before but in case you're skipping

around, I'll say it again. Locate the clitoris, one of the most important landmarks on a woman's body, at the front of the genital area, between the outer, fleshy lips. It will be quite small, possibly invisible, at the beginning, but as you continue foreplay it will become much more prominent.

- Stroke it very gently. Let her guide you as to how firmly to touch. I find that as I get more aroused I need much lighter touches. Pressure becomes almost painful.

- Slip only the tip of your finger inside her channel, then withdraw. Tease this way until she's squirming.

- Slowly insert an entire finger, then two and three if she's willing. Thrust and withdraw as a penis would during intercourse.

- Use the fingers of both hands, one on her clit and one inside.

A sixty-one-year-old woman wrote:
A man who can bring me off using only his hands is a pure joy. I've been with lots of men in my life and most of them thought that genital play was just foreplay. I can't come without a hand on my clit. It just doesn't happen. Sometimes I do it myself, but a guy who knows how to play with my clit while his penis is inside me is the best.

Actually, my husband of only three years knows how. He holds still at the moment of my climax and brings me off with his fingers. He says he can feel my orgasm on his cock.

I've had many perfect orgasms, ones that

couldn't get any better, all with manual stimulation, most with my husband.

A fifty-year-old man wrote:

It took me a lot of years to learn how to give a good hand job to my ladies. Is it a hand job when a guy gives it to a woman?

I've played and played and discovered that, while all women are different, and *vive la différence,* the same basics seem to work for most: lots of playing, sliding through folds, and waiting until she's really wet to enter her. Guys, be patient. It can be pure joy to watch her face contort and her body writhe when she comes. It's really nice for me to do it with my hands so my body's not involved yet. I especially love to wait until she thinks she's coming down, then ram my hard cock into her and make her climax again.

A forty-year-old man wrote:

An old-fashioned hand job is an integral component of my marriage, although most times it would be a stretch to classify our hand play as old-fashioned. Beyond being one of the most reliable methods of ensuring my wife's climax, it also adds some nice, quick variation to our lovemaking.

One of my favorite things to do is get my wife off while we're driving in our car. Though not particularly well suited for short commutes, there's nothing like sliding my hand in between my lover's thighs on some endless stretch of highway. If she immediately jumps or laughs at my initial touch, I know that the time isn't right. But if my hand is welcomed by a subtle relaxation of her thighs, I know that my wife is wanting, and I'm more than happy to oblige.

Our first "highway hand-job" experience was while driving to our honeymoon destination the morning after our wedding. It progressed out of some mutual heavy petting over the top of each other's clothes, to my rubbing my wife's swollen clit under her panties as she sat in the passenger's seat. I'll never forget spreading her engorged labia to gain access to her hard nubbin while she proceeded to grind her wet pussy against my fingers. The visual of her unbuttoning her top so she could pleasure her own breasts almost made me cream my jeans. After only a few minutes of this I pulled off the road, and we rubbed each other to orgasm right there in the front seat.

Some five years later, we never fail to take advantage of a lengthy drive without our children (which is unfortunately rare). If there are any tips that I could pass along to people interested in trying this, I'd leave you with two important points:

1. Nothing beats the ease of access afforded by a skirt.
2. Three words: Front-clasp bra.

Note: Beware of distracted driving! As an EMT I've responded to too many accidents where the driver of a car was not devoting full attention to the road—including several as described above. Talk about embarrassing—and potentially very serious!

Intermammary Intercourse

As we all know, making love with a woman can take many forms. One that's frequently overlooked is intermammary intercourse, usually known by its slang term, tit fucking. Many couples play this way, and both parties can get a great deal of pleasure from it. It's also a good way to make love when vaginal intercourse isn't possible.

How to Give It

A twenty-eight-year-old man wrote:
> The girl that I have been dating for the last month slept over at my house last week and we had our first sexual experience together. The sex, however, didn't include penile–vaginal contact.
>
> We were in my bed nude with the covers back and I lay on my back. Sue straddled me and began rubbing her breasts on my chest. She is a tall woman with long legs, perky breasts, and small hard nipples that poke out like new pencil erasers. Her breasts are small but firm, and as she rubbed her nipples along my body I could feel my excitement level rising.
>
> She rubbed her breasts on the inside of my thighs and on my penis, and when my penis became stiff she rubbed her breasts on it very lightly. She kept the rubbing going for over ten minutes, and when the pre-cum began to flow her nipples got wet, which made the contact more slippery and thus more exciting.

All of a sudden Sue held my penis by the shaft and began to rub her breasts and nipples vigorously on the head of my penis until I ejaculated in powerful spurts. When she rose over me a small drop of semen was slowly dripping from her nipple and this nearly drove me crazy. I flipped her over and licked and sucked her breasts and pussy until she came too.

A forty-one-year-old man wrote:

I've discovered an interesting variation on breast sex that others may want to try. I doubt if it is an original idea, but last night my honey and I discovered or invented something that really enhanced one of our favorite bedroom pastimes.

We both really get off on tit fucking and do it on a regular basis. Last night I had an idea, and after telling her about it she really got into it. We took an old bra of hers that is a size too small. First we cut away most of the cups so her nipples and most of her tits were exposed. Then we trimmed around the bottom and top of what remained around the cleavage so there was only enough of the material left to keep the cups attached to each other. The beauty of this modified bra is that neither of us has to use our hands to hold her tits together while my cock is slipping back and forth between them. This leaves both of us with our hands free to do anything else with them we would like. Simply apply your preferred lubricant, slide your stiff dick into the convenient opening, and go to town!!

A twenty-nine-year-old woman wrote:

I have always been well endowed (38DD) so I am well aware of how men like to, to put it bluntly, tit fuck. Like you see in the movies, it is best if you use oil of some type. I have done it in many positions, but I like the "on my back" position the best. I squeeze my breasts together and pinch my nipples while my husband fucks them. I prop my head up on some pillows so I can occasionally suck the head of his cock when it thrusts up through my cleavage. This is a great way to please my husband when I am otherwise "out of commission," but that is not the only time we do it. By the way, it does a lot for me too!

A forty-five-year-old woman wrote:

Breast fucking is very sensual. It is such a turn-on for me to know that I can make my husband come with just my breasts and nothing else. Of course, it seldom is nothing else!

I love to run my tongue around the head of his cock when he thrusts. Some sort of lubricant is a must, but for all you women who are nursing, forget the oils. When I was nursing my children, I would always have tremendous milk leakage during sex. I can tell you from experience that breast milk is a great lubricant for tit fucking! And it's right there where you need it, too! He would get hard *milking* me and rubbing it on his cock and between my engorged tits. It pleasured both of us!

CONDIMENTS

Chapter 6

ORAL SEX

NOW THAT WE'VE COVERED THE BASICS, THE filling for our sexual sandwich, let's take some time and talk about all the things you can add to spice up your meal: the salt and pepper, mustard, relish, and ketchup of lovemaking.

Oral sex is a singular pleasure. However, so many people are afraid of it, as I was years ago, that they shy away from trying it. Personally, I always thought there was a magic formula for pleasing a man—for giving good head. I was afraid to try, sure I didn't know the secret. Some women are just born knowing, I reasoned, or they are so intuitive that they know how to do it with only a little practice. I was also one of many who were, and still are, totally paralyzed by visions of Linda Lovelace in *Deep Throat*. I knew I couldn't do that, not with my overactive gag reflex, and if I couldn't then I'd never be any good at it. So I didn't do anything. On top of all that negative stuff, I was also afraid that it would smell bad and that, if my lover ejaculated, it would taste icky.

As for receiving, I knew there was an odor to my genitals, one I didn't like, and I assumed that a man would be turned off by my body's smell. So I made it known, in those nonverbal ways women have, that oral sex wasn't part of my lexicon. Alas.

Over the years I've learned a lot. There is no magic formula, and you don't have to be Linda Lovelace. Take your clues from your partner and relax. Just give it a try.

How to Give It for Her

Ladies, you don't have to suck on a man's genitals or take them deep into your throat to make him feel good. Take your time if you're new to this, and understand that even a little attention to his penis, just a bit of fellatio, makes most men crazy.

- Take off your rings and such and get your hair out of the way. It does look sexy in those porno movies for that woman to flip her long hair around, but in the real world it just gets in the way.

- Begin slowly, with kisses—light ones and heavy ones and all types between—on the shaft and on the head. If you're feeling brave, kiss his testicles.

- Flick the shaft or head of his penis with the tip of your tongue to get the feel and taste thing over with. Take your time, and if that's all you do for this encounter, then fine. Don't worry; you have time to make all of him all of yours.

- Move on to licks, like an all-day sucker. Use lots of saliva. Let him lead the way with his moans and purrs. Lick where he seems to like it and you'll quickly find that you enjoy it.

- Use your hands at the same time to stroke his shaft or cradle his testicles. Remember that a man's shaft can take pretty hard squeezes and prolonged rubbing.

- Stop every once in a while to tell him how sexy it all is. This also allows the tension to ebb a bit so you can build it up again.

- Once you decide to take his penis into your mouth, go slowly. You don't have to devour him, just suck lightly on the head while rolling your tongue around or flicking it. Take as much of him into your mouth as you're comfortable with and no more.

- Eventually, if you want, take the length of his penis in your mouth and breathe through your nose.

- If you want to spice things up further, add whipped cream, maple syrup, or whatever takes a while to lick off. Go farther by putting a small piece of ice in your mouth for a sexy surprise. Use your teeth lightly to change the sensation.

- Take your time. Eventually he'll let you know when he's ready to jump your bones.

- Gaze at him while you do it. It will excite him and arouse you by watching his pleasure.

A forty-year-old woman wrote:

Most women I know think of oral sex as a chore or, at best, a gift unselfishly given to a man with no pleasure received in return. I am not one of these women.

I have always taken great pleasure from licking, caressing, and sucking a man into ecstasy. Nothing gets me wetter and hotter than the feeling of a big hard cock sliding in and out of my mouth. When discussing oral sex with other women I usually find myself hushed by skeptical comments and doubting looks. I am using this opportunity to speak my piece.

Ladies, if you don't enjoy oral sex, try this approach. Stop focusing on what's going on in your mouth and start paying attention to what is happening to your man's body. Feel how hard his cock gets the instant it touches your lips. Look at the uncontrollable expressions of ecstasy on his face. Listen to the exciting sounds of pleasure he makes. And last but definitely not least enjoy the intensely satisfying sexual experience he will give you in return.

A fifty-one-year-old man wrote:

I prefer to lie propped up on pillows, to watch my lady make love to me with her mouth. I love to watch her slowly lick the shaft from its base to the tip, paying special attention to the tender nerve endings just below the head. Then, as I watch, she sucks my testicles into her mouth, one at a time, gently rolling them around with her tongue. She returns to licking the shaft, wetting it all over, and sucking it deep into her throat.

She will often open her eyes just to see the effect she has on me, and often she gets excited to the point where she will turn around placing her mound on my face and start rubbing, insisting that I return her favors. I always do, gladly, of course.

At this point in time my wife does not enjoy it if I come in her mouth. She either shoots my seed between her large breasts, or mounts me just in time to let me finish deep inside her, and that's just fine with me.

Oral Sex

A fifty-seven-year-old man wrote:

When a woman goes down on me I like to feel as if she is worshiping my penis. I like her to smother my penis and balls with kisses, to lightly rub my hard cock against her face, and to rub the head of my penis back and forth between her lips, lightly touching me with her tongue but not yet taking me in her mouth.

Since the physical sensation and psychological excitement of having a woman take me in her mouth is so intense, I like a woman to take her time and not let me come too quickly. She can do this by spending a lot of time playing before she takes me in her mouth. I like her to lick the entire length of my penis, from base to tip. This feels so good I would love her to do it for hours! It also feels good to have her turn her head sideways and suck on me like an ear of corn.

I like to have special attention played to my balls, gently of course. She can kiss them, lick them, gently bring them into her mouth one at a time, and lift them so she can lick right behind them. Wow, I love that! When she places the tip of her tongue right behind my balls and licks with one long slow stroke across my scrotum and up the penis to the tip, I am in heaven.

I also love it when a woman watches for the first small amount of pre-come ooze out of the tip of my penis, and then licks it off while looking me in the eyes. It is like my semen is so precious she doesn't want to waste a drop.

When she finally takes me in her mouth, I love her to cup my balls in one hand and have her other hand around the base of my penis. Now she can experiment with moving back and forth, flicking her tongue against the sensitive underside of my cock, and taking me as deep into her mouth as is comfortable for her. When I get close to coming, I like her to stop and go back to some of the earlier foreplay techniques like licking me or playing with my balls, just to make the experience last.

When she finally lets me come, I love her to make a soft purring sound and to suck every last drop out of me. This makes me feel totally loved and accepted, and to want to do the same for her!

A *twenty-seven-year-old woman* wrote:
I've read a lot about oral sex and I think that I must be just weird. I love to perform on men. No, that is not the weird part. What is really odd is the fact that I can orgasm from it. If I take his penis deep into my mouth, stroking with my tongue, I can eventually bring myself to orgasm. I've had several boyfriends tell me that it is not possible, but when the time is right I show them.

How to Get It for Him

Guys, you've probably just read what I wrote for her, so the primary rule is *Help her*. Show her in every way you can how and where and what feels best. Do lots of moaning. Tell her how great she's making you feel.

Don't be threatening. I remember a letter from a woman whose head was held during her first efforts at oral sex. She never did it again. If you want to touch your lady while she's learning, cup the sides of her face. Don't tangle your fingers in her hair, as sexy as this seems. It can make a woman feel trapped.

I suggested to the woman in the last paragraph that she tie her current lover's hands so she was in complete charge. Not a bad idea.

Then there's the swallowing thing. Guys, let that go, at least in the beginning. Assure her that you'll let her know when you're close to coming so she doesn't have to worry about you ejaculating in her mouth. No surprises! You'll run the risk of turning her off so she'll be reluctant to try again. If, eventually, you want to broach the subject, ask her whether she'd like to try watching you ejaculate. Then you can advance to the cum shots they get in the porn movies. Can swallowing be far behind? Just take your time and talk with her at every juncture. And if she never swallows, let it go. It's unimportant in the world of great sex.

A twenty-two-year-old woman wrote:

> I absolutely, positively adore giving my boyfriend a blow job. I used to hate the idea of fellatio because I felt it was an uneven power play that benefited the man more than the woman. That was until I met my current boyfriend.
>
> I love him very much and the love I have for him extends to all parts of him, especially his cock. The look on his face as I take him in my mouth, the feel of his hand on my head as he gently guides me, the soft moans and whimpers that he makes as I lick, suck, and nibble on him, all drive me wild. I get very aroused when I give him head, which never used to happen to me.
>
> My first two experiences with oral sex were distasteful. The first man had the indecency to come in my mouth without warning while trying to shove his penis down my throat. I gagged pretty badly and I was sick to my stomach for hours afterward. The second guy was always beg-

ging for it, and since I knew he didn't love me, I felt like a prostitute. Performing on him left me feeling used.

My new boyfriend is a wonderful and caring human being who originally objected to oral sex because he thought that it objectified women. He was quite adamant that I not go down on him. One evening, just to be stubborn, I told him to close his eyes and pretend like it wasn't happening, and did it over his protests. He found that he loved it. And, to my surprise, I found that I loved it too.

I firmly believe that a guy has to taste right for me to give him head. The only man whose taste I have craved has been my boyfriend, and that says something about our relationship. Not a waking hour passes that I do not contemplate the delicious flavor of his pre-come, and the smooth and firm texture of his glans, even the musky taste of his testicles. I've caused him great consternation by unzipping his pants, pulling out his cock, and going down on him during movies or while he was on the phone with his parents. He says I'm a menace to a man's sanity.

Ladies, if it doesn't taste right then chances are that you're blowing the wrong man. Find someone whose taste you lust after and more than likely that's a man you'll want to keep around. This goes for all you gentlemen, too.

As for taste, women have written that a man's taste is affected by what he eats. One woman wrote that if your guy eats peppermint or cinnamon, his semen tastes of it. Others swear by fruit juice, particularly pineapple. As I'm sure you already know, experimenting can be fun.

A thirty-nine-year-old woman wrote:

My ex-husband loved oral sex. He loved to give as much as receive. When we were first married it took me a while to give him head for the first time but he knew all the wonderful ways to convince me. Mostly he just told me how much he'd like it if I'd just try. He also never tried to push it on me.

One day I tried and found that I liked the feel of his soft cock getting hard in my mouth. The only thing that I could not do was swallow. I tried but I just couldn't do it. He understood and never tried to force me to do it.

Since my divorce I have had a couple of affairs, and I quickly let the guy know that I could not swallow. I was surprised at how many men were very understanding about this. Maybe someday I will be able to swallow but until then, I will give my man all the pleasure of oral sex that I can.

Ladies, don't worry about not being able to swallow. If you treat your man like he is the best thing since sliced bread, then not being able to swallow won't matter. Go for it!

How to Give It for Him

Men, if you're able to perform good cunnilingus, you'll never want for great sex. More importantly, eventually, perfect orgasms will be possible for both of you. If you've always wanted to know the secret to performing it, there is none. Sorry. Every woman is different, and there's no magic formula.

I think women are even more varied in what they like than men.

Just to make it more complicated, different strokes and licks feel good at different times. Early on, you can be a bit firmer, but as she gets more aroused, those firmer touches might be too much. Explore. That's what I like best, and she probably does too.

You should now be able to locate her clitoris. Touch it lightly and gauge your strokes by her reactions. If she seems to pull away a little, don't be discouraged. It might just mean she wants a lighter touch.

These tongue strokes work for many, so give them a try:

- Lick from the vagina to the tip of the clitoris gently.

- Try delving deeply into the grooves on each slide, long slow strokes first on one side, then the other. You might discover that one side is much more sensitive and arousing than the other.

- With the point of your tongue, swirl clockwise, then counterclockwise.

- Try gently sucking on her clit and gauge her reactions. More? Less? It's up to you to judge.

- When you think she's ready, you can insert the pointed tip of your tongue into her vaginal canal. For me, I prefer a finger or toy since it makes more of a statement and by then I'm ready for bigger stuff.

- Try humming slightly to make your lips and tongue vibrate.

- Don't let your hands be idle either. Cup her buttocks. Slide a finger inside.

- Don't hesitate to play with toys while you use your mouth and hands. Sliding a large dildo into her while your mouth does its dance can be fabulous.

- Explore and enjoy.

A forty-year-old man wrote:

My girlfriend and I dated for several years before I finally learned how to properly perform oral sex on her. I think many guys make the mistake of trying to pleasure their women in the way that they would like to be pleasured. That's a mistake. Women require different attention from men.

To begin with, my girlfriend had a hard time coming to grips with the fact that I wanted to put my mouth on her vagina. She was used to sucking me until I came, but she somehow thought that licking her vagina was less appealing. Ha!

To get her used to the idea, I made her shower before I first performed on her. This got around her perception that her genitals were somehow unappealing. Once she felt clean I could get her to relax while licking her but she did not have an orgasm. She was still extremely self-conscious. The next step was to let her know how much I wanted to make her come with my face in between her legs. I picked a night when we were going out and I began by telling her how much I wanted to give her oral sex. During the evening I constantly whispered into her ear how much I wanted to eat her wet pussy. I told her how I would not be satisfied until her wetness soaked my face. Needless to say we went home early that night because her whole outlook was changing. Whereas before she had tolerated my tongue's exploration, that night she craved it. As I licked her her hips went crazy and she forced herself into my mouth. Eventually her gyrations turned into orgasm and she came over and over again until my entire face was soaked with her juices.

Our sex life took a new direction once she became confident that I really enjoyed burying my face in her pussy. At that point I really learned how to satisfy her orally. Instead of trying to make her come in a hurry I slowed down and licked her entire pussy over and over until I could identify which part was making her feel good, which varies each time. Sometimes she wants my tongue on her clit only, sometimes she likes long slow licks, and at still other times can't get off without a couple of my fingers inside her. The key is that I now know not to hurry her, but to respond to her body. And all of this is pointless unless I let her know how much I want her ahead of time. A simple note in the morning or a phone call during the day telling her how much I want her makes all the difference in the world.

A forty-year-old man wrote:

I really love performing oral sex on a woman. I can remember fantasizing about it long before I ever had a chance to try it.

I find a woman's pussy to be an almost magical and mysterious source of excitement and pleasure. It feels so good around my penis that sometimes I just want to go down there to try and unlock its mysteries. I love the anticipation of kissing my way down a woman's stomach. I love a woman's soft silky pubic hair, especially when it is neatly trimmed into an alluring triangle, seeming to point the way to go for pleasure.

Sometimes I will wrap my arms around my wife and just rest my face on her pubic hair. It is comforting for some reason, to be so near the life-giving power of a woman. I also like to gently rub my face against her; it is as if she is scent-marking me as hers.

I am incredibly turned on by the way a woman's pussy looks. I love a woman's outer lips; they seem to exude raw sexual power. I remember the first time I really saw a woman from behind; she was on her knees and had her face down on a pillow, her head resting on her arms with her nice ass up in the air waiting for me to enter her. Her outer lips were quite visible to me, as was her anus and vaginal opening, and the view turned me on like you wouldn't believe. I like how soft the lips are. I like to look at them, feel them with my fingers, kiss them, lick them, and finally pull them into my mouth and suck on them like a baby.

I also like to spread the outer lips to get to her inner ones. It is like looking through the petals of a soft, pink, sweet flower. I like running my tongue up her inner lips to find the hidden prize of her clitoris at the top. It makes me feel good that I know exactly where her clitoris is, and what type of gentle but steady licking rhythm will drive her crazy. I also love knowing that I can make a woman wet with excitement. The scent and taste are mild, pleasant, and, for me, totally intoxicating. I really think women taste good. It is pure sex to taste a woman, and any man who doesn't is really missing something.

I enjoy going down on a woman from many positions. The traditional, with her lying on her back and me lying on my stomach between her legs, is very nice. It is also fun to lift her legs and rest them over my shoulders as I eat her. I also like to push her knees up with her heels against her buttocks so she is more exposed to my explorations. I think the best position is with her lying on the edge of the bed and me sitting on the floor in front of her. I can see everything this way. She can also sit in a comfortable living room chair, heels against her buttocks. My wife and I tried this recently and it was very erotic because I could stare into her eyes lovingly as I licked her. This is probably one of the only positions that enables the woman to see what is happening. It also makes it easy to insert a finger into her pussy as I'm eating her.

Another very erotic position is for me to lie on my back, and have her kneeling over me and slowly lower her pussy to my face. Having a woman "sit on my face" is so amazing. When she is smothering me with her pussy I forget about everything else in the world. I can look up at her breasts and face and see that I'm giving her so much pleasure that she can barely stay on top of me. I even like the feeling when she gets so aroused that her juices run down my face and neck. When she comes she practically falls over.

I have also found it fun to begin kissing my wife's neck, nibbling my way down her back to her buttocks, kissing and gently biting her beautiful ass and thighs, and trying to get my tongue to her pussy from this angle. I sometimes put my arms around her waist and pull her up so she is sticking her ass in the air and I get to her pussy that way. I can't really make her come like that because I can't reach her clitoris, but it is still sexy.

Of course the other wonderful oral sex experience is sixty-nine. Not being able to see anything but her sex really makes for a focused sexual experience. It has the same "smother me with your beautiful pussy" quality as having a woman sit on you, with the added benefit of feeling her warm body against mine and her face against my genitals or my hard cock in her mouth. She generally takes me out of her mouth well before she comes because it is too hard to concentrate on both giving and receiving!

I like to reach my arms around her and firmly grasp her buttocks and separate them as I eat her. It is an amazing feeling to make her come this way, and it is often quicker than other methods because my tongue is naturally positioned against her clitoris. Since she is resting on my face, I don't just lick her clitoral area, but I draw her lips and clit into my mouth and move my tongue against her. I love it when she comes and then collapses with her hot wet pussy right onto my chest. All I see is her sex and the taste and scent that envelop me are those of an aroused woman whom I just made come.

A fifty-one-year-old man wrote:
The most important thing about being good at performing oral sex (for a man or a woman) is the enthusiasm that comes from really liking it. For instance, while of course I want to give my partner pleasure, I really do love eating pussy and I would do it just for my own pleasure. I make sure she knows I love it, not just by doing it, but by telling her how beautiful her pussy is, how I love tasting

her, how her scent drives me crazy, and I even
make *mmmmm* sounds so she will feel like she is a
delicious dessert.

How to Get It for Her

Ladies, my advice to you is not very different from my advice
above for him. Be as demonstrative as you can. Show him and tell
him exactly what you enjoy. Keep the comments positive. "I love it
when you do it just that way." "Oooh, soft touches feel so right."
"You've got a great mouth." If he's doing something that doesn't feel
good, try "I love it when you do . . . rather than . . ." Keep it positive
but remember, you're teaching him just the way you'd like him to
teach you.

Let's begin with a few letters about why, then move on to
descriptions of how to both give and get. These letters speak for
themselves. From eating to doing a sixty-nine, from going down to
giving blow jobs, it seems many people can't get enough.

A forty-six-year-old man wrote:

My wife and I have been married twenty-two years
and in the past four or five years we have really
started enjoying mutual oral sex. I've been eating
her for quite a long while. I really love to pleasure
her, and since she has a very sensitive clit, she loves
it too. During the last few years she has really gotten into giving me oral sex too, and it really excites
both of us.

I love watching her and what she does, and she
loves the thrill of me seeing her with my cock in
her mouth. Instead of thinking this is bad, as she
did for much of our married life, she looks at this
as another way of lovemaking. We particularly love

to do a sixty-nine, during which we each pleasure the other.

Anyone not doing this with their partner is really missing out on something beautiful if it is done with passion and feelings.

A forty-one-year-old woman wrote:

My husband and I love oral sex and we indulge almost every time we make love. However, I hate sixty-nine. We tried it when we first made love, and for a while that's the position we used, with me sucking him while he did me. Finally I got brave enough to ask for one activity at a time. I told my husband that I lost a lot by not being able to concentrate on the pleasures he was giving me or I was giving him. Funny, it turned out he had the same feelings.

Now we do one thing at a time, and boy, do we do it well!

A twenty-eight-year-old man wrote:

I go down on my wife nine times out of ten when we make love. I fell in love with eating pussy when we were teenagers. She loves having me work her clit and finger her at the same time. She will tell me "come on" when she wants my cock.

As for receiving, I love to have my cock sucked. When my wife sucks me off, she holds me on the edge of orgasm for what seems like forever. Recently, after plenty of oral, she gave me a straight hand job. My orgasm was as intense as any I have ever had and when I came she did not quit stroking. Wow, what a feeling.

My advice? Ladies, try lots of ways to give

pleasure. Men, always offer the lady the option for oral. Then let your partner be your guide.

A thirty-seven-year-old woman wrote:

I am a lady who loves cunnilingus so much that I can't get enough of having my clitoris licked and sucked on. I love everything about oral. I like being licked and sucked all over my pussy. I am so lucky to have found a man, my boyfriend and soon-to-be husband, who loves oral sex just as much as I do.

I particularly love it when I wake up in the middle of the night and find him eating my pussy. Often my wake-up call in the morning is his tongue in my cunt licking and playing with me. He makes me so horny when he sticks his finger in my cunt, takes it out, and licks it before he goes down on me. He will not stop eating and sucking me until I come in his mouth a couple of times. In a way I'm really envious. I can only suck him and have him come once while he can bring me to orgasm four or five times. He says that his pleasure is knowing that he can make me come over and over again.

For all you ladies out there, don't stop looking. Out there is a man who would love to eat you as much as mine likes and enjoys eating me. I wish you all the best!

A thirty-eight-year-old woman wrote:

I had never tried oral sex on a guy until last fall with my lover and I never knew what joy I was missing. My ex-husband thought oral sex was disgusting, so I had no idea about how to give my new lover pleasure this way. I knew I wanted to try, however, and of course, he was all for it. He showed me what he liked and I tried lots of things I read in books and saw in porno flicks. And, of course, we practiced a lot. If his reactions are any judge, I have learned to do it really well.

Oh, my God—just knowing how much he enjoyed it was a turn-on in itself. I can come just from sucking my lover and, when he reciprocated, well I thought I had died and gone to heaven.

A forty-seven-year-old man wrote:

I am a man who loves oral sex. I love receiving it but I enjoy giving it even more. I had one thirty-year-old lover recently tell me that she loved to receive oral sex but she had never climaxed from it. That was the only challenge I needed. I succeeded in making her quiver and scream and fall limp with my face buried snugly in her sex. It is so intimate, being lost between my lover's thighs and giving her attention from my lips and tongue. I could make love like that forever. Feeling her respond by tightening her thighs around my head and bucking her pussy into my face as she reaches orgasm is the sex I live for.

A thirty-two-year-old man wrote:

Much of the reluctance around oral sex seems to be about body image. People who are embarrassed by their genitals aren't interested in exposing them or enjoying their partner's. It is as if the genitals are some foreign part of the body, not really part of the person. You can't expect individuals to enjoy oral sex until they can appreciate the beauty of their own body. The first step toward giving and receiving good oral sex is a delight and curiosity in your own and your partner's sexual equipment.

It doesn't matter what you look like. Particularly for the ladies, act like your genitals are a real gift to your partner and you'll enjoy a great sex life.

Chapter 7

BLINDFOLDS, STRIPPING, AND OTHER NAUGHTINESS

Blindfolds

WHY BLINDFOLD YOUR PARTNER? REMOVING ONE sense makes the mind concentrate on all the others. Your partner will listen more carefully to the movements of your body, your moans of pleasure. Smell and taste will be sharper. Unexpected touches of all kinds, from the stroke of a cotton pad or a feather to the scratch of sandpaper, will seem more intense. Changes of temperature, like the feel of a cup of warm water or the chill of an ice cube, will increase the thrill.

As with many of the games we'll talk about, blindfolding your partner requires a level of trust that you and your partner must achieve before you can play. Make sure that you two have agreed that *stop* means *stop* at any time during lovemaking. If you want to be able to say *stop* playfully without your partner actually ceasing activities, agree on a safe word—say, *marshmallow* or *mushroom*—that will say "Really, stop! Now!"

It's not necessary to purchase a ready-made blindfold. Blindfolds can be made from virtually anything, from the belt of a cotton robe to a necktie. If you truly want your partner not to be able to see anything, place a cotton ball on each eyelid before tying on the material. That way your lover won't be able to peek out beneath as you used to do when playing pin the tail on the donkey when you were a kid. However, if your partner's a bit reticent to try this, you might make the blindfold loose at first and allow a little peeking, just for reassurance.

One delicious technique is to leave your blindfolded partner alone for a short while, then enter the room and putter around. You'll have your lover thinking that all kinds of delicious things are going to happen, and then you can make them happen.

Let's see how ordinary folks like you use blindfolds as part of their sex play. This first letter is a great how-to guide.

How to Give It

A forty-year-old man wrote:

>Blindfolding is one of our favorite ways to play, so maybe this will inspire somebody. As somebody who loves to blindfold my partner (and to be blindfolded by her), I'm always trying to come up with fresh approaches on how to make it even more enticing and fun.

>For example, let me tell you about a recent playdate we had together. It started when I told her to change her clothes and dress provocatively in boots, nylons, open crotch panties, and no bra. And of course last but not least, a blindfold. She knew that I was planning something delightfully different and thus her arousal began immediately.

Blindfolds, Stripping, and Other Naughtiness

She changed her clothes and sat on the edge of the bed thinking about what was to come. The anticipation makes it all the sweeter for both of us.

I made her wait for a few minutes then I took her by the hand and walked her downstairs to our front room. I had pushed back the furniture, spread a sheet on the floor, and added a couple of pillows. I put on soft music and closed the curtains. Actually, I didn't tell her that last part. I wanted her to relish the dangerous possibility that we might be seen.

I walked her to the middle of the room and told her to kneel with her hands behind her back. While she knelt there, I walked around her slowly, telling her that she was my sex toy and that I would spend the next hour mercilessly teasing and taunting her. Around her, I told her, were ten items. Without seeing the items, just by picking a number, she would select one at a time and then I would use it on her for up to five minutes. We only got through about half the items before she climbed atop me, panting, and finished the game. The items (and the planned use and her position for each) were:

1. Strawberries and grapes. I fed these to her— on her knees, with her hands behind her back.

2. Ice. I touched all her most sensitive parts as she lay on her back spread-eagled.

3. Orange halves and honey. I spread the honey on her breasts, then mopped it up with the orange. Messy but I had warm, wet

towels (in a baby bottle warmer) nearby to clean up before she selected the next item.

4. Whipped cream. I told her to drop her shorts and lie on her back, spread open. Then I smeared the luscious cream on all the obvious places, then licked it off.

5. A hairbrush. She got into a kneeling position and I massaged her scalp and pussy. Then I used the brush to give her one or two playful slaps by surprise.

6. Feathers. My lady is ticklish and enjoys being tickled as part of foreplay.

7. A vibrating glove. She lay on her stomach as I gave her a full-body massage. And I do mean full-body.

8. A piece of fur. I stroked her all over as she lay on her back.

9. Fragrant hot herb tea in a thermos. She sat cross legged as I served it to her, then she licked it from my fingers.

10. A piece of silk. She knelt and pulled her panties down to her knees. I gently rubbed the silk all over her skin for a minute, then used it to tie her hands together in front of her and just sat back and looked at her, telling her how lucky I was to have a part-ner as lovely and cooperative as she is.

A twenty-eight-year-old woman wrote:

I don't know whether I've ever had a perfect orgasm but I've had some pretty good ones. My husband is a very creative guy and we have had some amazing times together. I guess the best I can remember is the time he blindfolded me. Somehow being deprived of sight made everything better.

It began one evening when, I'll admit, we'd had a few beers and were feeling pretty experimental. He told me to go into the bedroom and wait for him. From the gleam in his eye I knew he had something kinky in mind, so I gladly obliged. I could hear him fussing around the house, then he came into the bedroom with a plastic bag full of stuff. "Why don't you get undressed," he said. I did. I'm not the most gorgeous thing going but the way he looks at me makes me feel sexy. Okay, I'll admit it, I was also horny as hell and couldn't wait to get my clothes off.

"Come here," he said and I walked up to him. It was sort of a kick being naked when he was completely dressed. He turned me around and I heard him get something from the bag. Then he blindfolded me with a kitchen towel. Of course I could see underneath, you know, like you used to when you played blindman's bluff.

He knows me too well. "Hang on a minute." He went into the bathroom and got some of those cotton balls I use to take off my makeup. He untied the blindfold and put the cotton over my eyes, then retied the towel. I couldn't see a thing. "Okay, just stand there," he said. It was amazing. I had been really excited before but now I was crazy.

My knees shook and I was sooo very wet. I never imagined I could be so hot without him ever touching me.

Anyway, I felt him come around to stand in front of me. I couldn't imagine what he was going to do, but he said, "Open your mouth." He'd obviously raided the fridge because he put a small piece of chocolate in my mouth. Then he kissed me. I couldn't figure out whether to chew or kiss him back. When he pulled away, I chewed quickly so I could tell him how aroused I was, but he put his finger over my lips. "Just enjoy," he said, his voice sexy and hoarse.

For the next five minutes I stood in our bedroom, naked and blindfolded, tasting. It was the most sensual thing I think I've ever done. He fed me everything from Cheerios to ice cream. I think the sexiest was the last, peanut butter. I licked and sucked it from his finger. Actually I enjoyed teasing him, swirling my tongue over his finger like giving oral sex to his cock. I guess I got to him because he picked me up and put me on the bed.

We have a silky spread and it felt all cold and slithery. I guess I never noticed how erotic that was until I couldn't see. While I waited for him to join me, I wriggled my bottom over the material. It was dynamite. He stretched out beside me and pressed the length of his naked body against mine. His cock was so hard and so hot against my hip that I couldn't wait. I grabbed him as his fingers played with my nipples, just the way I liked. I was afraid I'd climax before we ever did it.

Still blindfolded I straddled his hips and slowly lowered myself onto him. We'd done it in this position a few times before but this was the best. Without being able to see, he became just a cock that I could have whatever way I wanted. I did him slowly, then fast. I teased him by letting only a little inside, then backing off.

We must have done it for ten minutes, just getting higher and higher. Finally he said, "Shit, baby, I can't hold out much longer." So I stretched out over him and he rolled me over on my back. We both like it best in that position and he pounded into me like there was no tomorrow. I came then, my spasms lasting so long I thought I'd never come down. My whole body shook and I think I passed out for a short time. It was just the best ever.

Perfect orgasm? I don't know how it could have been any better.

A thirty-six-year-old man wrote:
The tie belts that accompany bathrobes make excellent ad hoc blindfolds. Just cover her eyes with the belt and tie it behind her head to secure it in place. If she is amenable to it, you can hold on to the ends and use them to guide her mouth for the best rhythm and penetration depth when she's kneeling in front of you performing fellatio.

How to Get It

A twenty-eight-year-old woman wrote:
This year my husband and I were very busy and it was finally Christmas Eve and he told me he had dozens of packages to wrap and needed my help.

Since some of them were for me and he didn't want me to see, he had a fiendish idea. He blindfolded me and then had me help him wrap my own presents—hold this, put your finger here, and so on. This was the first time I'd been blindfolded since I was a kid and I found it really arousing. By the time all the packages were wrapped, I was so hot I dragged my hubby up the stairs and we went at it. Since then, blindfolds have become part of lots of our playtimes.

Mirrors

While we're talking about sight, a word about mirrors. Have you ever watched yourself make love? It's dynamite. One more sensation to add to all the others.

How to Get It

A *thirty-one-year-old woman* wrote:

The most perfect orgasm I can ever remember was when I discovered that my husband of four years had positioned the mirror on my dresser so he could watch us while we made love. I hadn't realized it at the time but for quite a while he had been watching us. Here's what happened.

One evening I opened my eyes during lovemaking and noticed that his eyes were fastened on that mirror. It took only a glance to see what he could see. I froze and he knew he'd been caught.

We stopped and talked about it. He said it was a giant turn-on for him and suggested that it might be for me as well.

At first I was really repelled by the idea. I'm not too happy with my body and I couldn't imagine wanting to see myself the way he sees me. I like to think I'm beautiful, especially when we're doing it, but I know that it's my little fantasy. In reality, all I wanted to do was turn off the lights and go back to what we'd been doing, but he started to stroke me and get me excited. I sort of forgot the mirror until he said, "Look how beautiful you are when you're really hot."

Well, I looked. There I was, my hair all scrambled, my face flushed, my legs spread with my husband's hand working away. It was awesome. As I watched I got hotter and hotter until, when I watched him fucking me, I thought I'd come forever. Now I understand that he's not affected at all by my looks. It's me he wants, and now we both watch.

A twenty-nine-year-old man wrote:

Have you ever done it in the bathroom of a motel, on the counter, in front of that huge mirror? One night, my wife and I had traveled to another city for a wedding, and after the rehearsal dinner we were both pretty blitzed. I went into the bathroom to shower and she followed, talking about the couples and the party.

When I came out of the shower, there she was, wearing only a tiny bra and pair of panties, looking so scrumptious that I grabbed her and kissed her good. It took only a few moments for us both to

become really aroused so I sat her on the bathroom counter and turned her so she faced it. I
pressed my chest against her back and I slipped my
hands under her bra. As we watched I kneaded her
globes and tugged at her nipples.

One thing led to another and soon she was
naked, still facing the mirror, legs spread. We
stared, almost mesmerized, while I stroked her
pussy and rubbed my cock up and down the crack
of her ass. I tried to control our orgasms and managed to come just after she did.

Sadly, we've never done that again. I wonder
why not. Now that I've written this letter I think I'll
invite my lovely wife to spend a night with me in a
nearby motel.

Note: Mirrors on the ceiling have long been a sta-
ple of hedonistic hotels, and watching yourself and
your partner from above is a terrific turn-on. If
you're considering mirroring your ceiling, however, please be sure to have a professional do the
construction. If you do it yourself, one wrong
vibration and the entire thing might come down.
Take care.

Lingerie

Wearing sexy undies can be a turn-on not only for him but for you
too, ladies. Honest. Ed doesn't care what I wear under my clothes.
Sexy lingerie isn't a turn-on for him, so for a long time I wore serv-
iceable bras and cotton panties. Eventually I decided that I liked the
way I felt in something a bit more daring and so I bought a few lacy

bras and pairs of panties. I wish I could say that Ed gazed at me with lust the first time he saw me, but, alas, he still doesn't notice. I feel sexier, however, and that's what matters to me.

How to Get It for Her

Victoria's Secret stores are everywhere, and I'm sure you can find something that will arouse and entice. Victoria's Secret items are expensive, however, and might be a bit out of your price range. If so, try Wal-Mart. The makers of undies have discovered how much we women enjoy our sexy little items and have begun making really attractive and revealing things at very reasonable prices. Don't overlook the nighties, slips, and such too.

Victoria's Secret and Frederick's of Hollywood have delicious catalogs that by themselves can ignite an evening of passion. Just thumbing through one with your partner and getting suggestions on what to buy can really heat things up. And if you decide to buy something, it does arrive in a plain brown wrapper so you don't have to worry about what the mailman will think. Think of it as gift wrap and treat yourself and your partner.

There are also about a zillion sites on the Net that sell lingerie in all sizes. Please visit my Web site at www.joanelloyd.com and click over to my links page. There is an entire section devoted to purchasing items. I can't vouch for all of the sites listed, but I've never had a problem with credit cards or delivery with the ones I've used. They are in business to sell stuff, not rip you off.

Here's a different idea. Cut out the centers of the cups out of a few of those old bras and remove the crotch from old panties. Your partner will be in for quite a surprise when he undresses you.

A fifty-six-year-old man wrote:
> Wearing lingerie is definitely something that will
> spice up a nice evening of romance. From my

own experience I can say that the whole experience is better because wearing special items
shows that you care about yourself and your partner. There is so much lingerie out there that can
flatter even the most shy or uncomfortable
woman to the point that they can get a whole
new outlook on themselves.

Unfortunately the media has this annoying
habit of depicting the perfect woman as almost
anorexic and I can tell you that I prefer women
who don't look like those underweight, skin-and-
bones models. So for all you larger ladies out
there, do yourself and us men a favor and take
advantage of your voluptuous bodies and let us
enjoy them.

How to Give It

A thirty-year-old man wrote:

I like to see my lady in lingerie, and the more
diaphanous the better. I've bought her a couple of
baby doll outfits that she wears to bed sometimes
and I really love it when she rubs her silky self
against me. She also likes to sleep in an old cotton
T-shirt that's full of holes. I love that too, since it
doesn't hide much.

We both like it when she sits around the house
wearing not very much, and I always get horny
when she parades around in something revealing,
especially if she is feeling frisky and lets me know
it. We routinely tease each other to get things
started when we know we can't finish right then,

like during the Super Bowl (we weren't about to miss the "bowl"), but later, when we're back to getting it on, we are both really ready.

One last thing. I recently got her a couple of T-shirts that we both knew were too small for her and then cut them off right below her boobs so that it just barely keeps them hidden. I love it all!

A fifty-five-year-old man wrote:

I view lingerie and its use as sexual costuming. Most items of intimate apparel are designed to enhance sensation and entice during the ultimate in adult recreation.

Bras and panties worn daily by women generally don't count. However, garments like teddies, bustiers, crotchless panties, satin gloves, thigh-high nylons, and garter belts are all part of the costuming of sex, intended as part of role playing or just to heighten pleasure.

Personally, I prefer my wife to wear very elegant lingerie: long, flowing, satiny silky gowns with matching robes, elbow-length gloves, high-heeled slippers, dark, thigh-high nylons, and garter belts. I have purchased several such outfits over the years and am in constant search for more. These are generally not found in your ordinary franchised lingerie stores at the local mall. Rather, the kind of lingerie that I like is available from very fine specialty shops and is usually quite expensive. Many upscale boutiques sell the most elegant garments designed to help a woman feel sexy and perhaps act like a courtesan. The cost of a silk satin gown, long matching robe, gloves, mules (slippers), garter belt, and hose can run four to five hundred dollars, but it is worth the price—if one can afford it—because when a woman feels classically elegant, she turns on sexually.

My favorite scenario is to enter a candlelit room and watch my lady walk in wearing bright scarlet, or very light blue, or even virginal white, and sensuously strip, leaving on only her gloves, garter belt, hose, and high-heeled slippers. Nothing is quite as beautiful to me as seeing my wife's mons with her womanly cleft framed by the nylons and garter belt. Sometimes, when we are off to a major function involving business types or politicians, my wife will wear a very elegant dress and sometimes a garter belt and nylons with no panties. When she does this, she will take my hand and let me touch here bare thigh just above the stocking top and her uncovered womanhood. Or she will give me a sample taste of her passion from her fingertips. Needless to say, it has me in a state of arousal most of the night, and our conjugal union later is very intense.

A forty-six-year-old man wrote:

Sexy undies definitely make a difference to our lovemaking. My wife knows very well that if she is wearing a sexy lingerie set or garter belt she can get anything she wants. I am immediately turned on and at her mercy. It takes us hours to get her undressed, one erotic piece of clothing at a time. It is a slow process that turns us on so much that we sometimes have orgasm without intercourse. And of course when the lingerie is eventually tossed around the room we have the greatest sex imaginable.

A forty-year-old man wrote:

There is no greater turn-on in the whole wide world than seeing the love of your life in sexy underwear. For me the greatest fuck is the one where my lover is wearing nothing but black stockings and a garter belt. Even before the action begins, seeing her looking like a hooker excites me beyond measure and once the action starts the feel of the stockings brushing your back or ass is beyond description.

Some time ago my lover and I were on vacation and one evening the hotel room was distinctly chilly. She had made it to bed before me and when I climbed in I noticed—with a little disappointment—that she had put on a thick flannel nightie more suitable for her grandmother. Undeterred my hands went exploring anyway. To my delighted surprise, what did I find? Underneath she had on a pair of lacy crotchless panties! That was a huge turn-on and we still laugh together at the thought of it.

My all-time favorite, however, is a red teddy set with which she announces wordlessly exactly what she wants. Later, when we're making love she keeps everything on but the panties. To see my cock buried in her surrounded by red lace is pure bliss. Thank God for the warmth and closeness of lovemaking. I pity those poor souls who have never experienced the joy of being with a totally uninhibited lover.

A fifty-one-year-old man wrote:

Lingerie? That's an interesting topic because my lady does not have the perfect body. She has very large breasts, a large frame, and a belly. Years ago I would look at the magazines of skinny women with thongs or teddies on. I would then look at my wife and be disappointed, not in her body but in her reluctance to show it off.

Then I tried something new. I decided to buy what I wanted to see her in. What a difference this made almost immediately.

At first, when she opened the box, I think she was really upset. But eventually I convinced her to put on the teddy I had bought. Well, I think the look on my face when she came out of the bathroom surprised and delighted her. She didn't look like a skinny model, she looked like herself, but wrapped in something that said *I want you*. As time passed, she realized that I love her body because it's hers—and I like her to show it off.

Men out there, if this is your cup of tea by all means buy something for your lady that you'd like to see her wear. That way you get to see her in something you like on her and she feels more attractive knowing that you desire her.

A forty-four-year-old man wrote:
I have always liked the look of lingerie, especially the more "classic" pieces: corsets, teddies, garters, and hosiery. Black is the best color, because of the way it creates patterns of light and shadow on breasts, nipples, calves, ankles, and the vulva. My particular turn-on is seeing swollen, aroused labia pressed behind a sheer black panty or g-string. There's nothing like a pair of expensive, lace-top black sheer hose to bring out the

curves of a woman's legs, and there's something uniquely arousing about the upper arch of a woman's foot in a pair of high heels. Lingerie, like push-up or open-tip bras and crotchless panties, showcases the sexiest parts of the woman's anatomy.

Fine lingerie (sheer nylon, smooth silk, lace, ribbons, et cetera) enhances the female form and makes a particular statement to the man—that she cares enough to take the time to dress up for him. Lingerie only increases a man's level of arousal prior to any sexual activities.

How to Get It for Him

Sexy lingerie isn't only for women, you know.

Guys, there are lots of pouches, g-strings, and thongs that will not only show off your "equipment" but keep you mildly aroused all day as well.

A thirty-six-year-old man wrote:

When purchasing men's thongs and g-strings it is advisable to purchase the size above your normal size. For example, I have a thirty-two-inch waist but purchase size large in thongs and g-strings. I have found that my wife often does the same with her purchases for me. There's a particular site I enjoy. It's called www.Undergear.com, and I've found that it's the standard-bearer for men's briefs and swimwear. They provide excellent service, feature good-quality items, and have reasonable prices and an above-average selection that changes fairly often. This is a good store to find everything from everyday bikini briefs and thongs to silk g-strings and racy swimwear. Shop away, their products are a safe bet.

A *thirty-one-year-old man* wrote:

About two years ago I was doing my laundry and noticed how old my underwear had become. My Jockey shorts were about ten years old and my T-shirts were older than that and had quite a few holes. So I went to the Internet and logged on to a well-known department store and shopped for new underwear. I was amazed at the new styles available for men. I ordered a small variety to try out and see what I liked and what fit the best. I settled on Jockey nylon microfiber briefs and bikinis. I found that they ran small so had to buy a size larger than normal. Later I found 100 percent nylon briefs from Underwear Exchange at Target stores. These run true to size, but I still wear a size larger since I've discovered that I like a loose comfortable fit and I think they look sexier a little baggy. I bought some thongs that I wear while lounging around the house and on weekends while shopping for groceries and running errands. You must practice proper hygiene, but thongs feel great and are very sexy. Calvin Klein's nylon microfiber thongs and DKNY's flex thongs are the best. Again, I buy one size larger and enjoy the looser fit.

Guys! These are panties for men pure and simple, so go buy some for yourself and enjoy and stay out of your wife's panty drawer. You'll love the new feel and your mate will enjoy your new look.

How to Give It for Her

Ladies, as you've seen, guys like the feel of sexy undies too. If you give your lover a pair of satin shorts, or some of your silky panties, to wear beneath his business suit, the slippery feel of that slick material will have him thinking of the night to come all day. Tell him that you get really hot thinking of what he's wearing and how hard it makes his cock.

You might try gift-wrapping a pair of really naughty undies and putting them in his briefcase, with a warning to open in private. He can then change at work and wear them on the trip home. I hope he doesn't exceed the speed limit.

Stripping

I thought I'd include a few letters about stripping—for both men and women.

How to Give and Get It

A forty-eight-year-old woman wrote:
> After my husband and I had been married for sev-
> eral years our sex life was getting a bit dull. We sat
> down and talked about it and we asked each other
> whether there was anything we've wanted but
> never had the nerve to ask. We'd had a few beers
> so we were more open than we might have been at
> another time.
>
> Anyway, my husband said he'd always wanted

me to strip for him. I was shocked, not because the idea of stripping turned me off but because I don't have a great body. I've had four kids in a previous marriage and thought I was droopy, flabby, and full of stretch marks. He didn't care, he wanted me to do it. He didn't pressure me; he just mentioned it and then let the subject drop.

I thought about it for several weeks and decided that I wanted to make him happy, even if it made me a bit uncomfortable. We get the Playboy Channel on our dish so I secretly watched a few movies and one short film that showed strippers. Interesting. Of course they were gorgeous with slender, shapely bodies but my husband had asked me to do it. What the hell, I thought, I'd do it for him.

Having made the decision, I gave a lot of thought to what I should wear. I decided on a long-sleeve blouse so I could unbutton the buttons slowly and erotically, a short skirt with stockings, a garter belt I bought at a discount store, and a pair of high-heeled shoes I found in the back of my closet. I wanted to wear gloves like they do in the movies—you know, peel them off one at a time— but I was too embarrassed to be that blatant.

Well, one evening I did it. I told my husband to put some music on the CD player then sit on the sofa while I went into the bathroom and changed. I was terrified when I walked into the living room but my husband must have figured out what I was doing and, as I began, he clapped his hands and cheered me on like they do in the strip shows. He actually whistled. That gave me courage and such pleasure to know he was enjoying what I did. I made a few wrong moves and the zipper on my skirt got stuck but we didn't care. Even laughing was sexy.

Now I strip for him often. We use Monopoly money and he stuffs bills in my g-string, then I use the cash to buy sexual activities from him. It costs a thousand dollars for a full-body massage (and I do mean full-body) and I can earn that from one strip show.

Ladies, do it. He's not looking for one of those supermodels. He wants you!

Bravo. I couldn't have said it better myself.

A thirty-nine-year-old man wrote:

I have always wanted to make stripping, both for her and me, part of our lovemaking but making it happen takes some alcohol and a little luck. Eventually we found a game that helps.

My girlfriend and I both have a penchant for brightly colored underwear so I suggested a simple guessing game on one of our evenings together. She had made some comment about doing different things in the bedroom and elsewhere so my suggestion did not seem out of place. The basic idea was to guess the color of the other's panties. We would name colors alternately until one was correct. The winner could choose either to undress the other or to ask the other to do a striptease.

When she particularly wanted to win, she rigged the result. For example, on one occasion she removed all except one color of mine while I was out of my room that evening. The next day, when I came to select a color, there was only one. I should say that I wouldn't want to play this game if I had any heart problem as the anticipation really tends to build.

I've always loved watching her strip and I enjoy stripping for her. I love watching her face as I take off my clothes. However, sometimes she'll opt for undressing me if she wins. If you've never been undressed by a lover with talented hands, you haven't lived.

Chapter 8

TOYS

TOYS ARE A GREAT ADDITION TO A BEDROOM aimed at arriving at the perfect orgasm. They don't have to be purchased at a store. Lots of ordinary things can be fun if you can be a bit creative.

A forty-year-old man wrote:

> When my wife and I travel, I sometimes pack a "kit" for the motel bedroom. It has three of my favorite compact discs and a small player, some personal lubricant (I'm using one called Wet Platinum, which works just wonderfully), and two scarves that work for blindfolds, restraints, et cetera. I keep a few slender candles that I can light for ambience, or use for dildos if we get into that mood. I also try to gather a few to-go menus from the hotel lobby for some nearby restaurants, so when we're tired and hungry afterward we can indulge. Sometimes I order something really decadent when we arrive and feed it to her as part of

foreplay. We are not allowed napkins—we have to use our tongues.

A *forty-two-year-old man* wrote:

My wife and I have only tried a couple of things. We have a small vibrator, which I love to use on her or watch her use on herself and bring herself to orgasm. Here's an interesting idea. On occasion we've used a balloon, the long thin kind, slightly filled with warm water. It works a little like a dildo, but I can squeeze and release the part that is outside of her, which forces the water in and out. She goes crazy!

A *thirty-eight-year-old man* wrote:

I don't know whether you'd consider our bedroom a toy, but we do. We've arranged it so we can play some of our favorite games. We've filled the room with pillows of various shapes and sizes. Some I put under her hips, some I kneel on. Once we piled every one we owned on the bed and made love in the crowd.

We fastened long pieces of clothesline we got at the supermarket to the legs of our bed and we tuck them under the mattress for secrecy. When we want them, of course, they are already attached and ready for bondage play. In addition, since we enjoy an evening of tying or being tied, we have several plant hooks embedded in the ceiling. Most of the time we use them to hang plants. However . . .

A *thirty-one-year-old woman* wrote:

My husband and I are always on a very tight budget

and can't afford to buy sex toys. That doesn't stop our play, however. It began one evening when we decided to play a game of *what if*. This one was "what if we had five hundred dollars to spend in a sex store." We connected to the Net and started to dream.

We looked at the dildos and I started to think that some household things might do just as well. Now we use a cucumber or thick carrot, well washed, of course, or a candle. We now have ones of varying thicknesses, depending on my mood.

When he told me he wanted to try a cock ring I remembered the roll of Velcro I had used for making a costume for one of my kids. We experimented and finally had something that worked pretty well. My husband fooled around with a few clothespins and loosened the pinch so they made good nipple clamps.

Well, now we wander through catalogs and sites improvising as we go. Somehow the thought and planning just add to the fun.

There are so many different varieties of sex toy that I suggest you let your fingers do the walking through a large adult-product catalog or Web site. Adam & Eve, Good Vibrations, and Xandria are a few of the big ones, but there are thousands of Web sites out there. If you like, visit my Web site at www.joanlloyd.com, click over to my list of links, and visit any one of them. Merely wandering through such a virtual store with your partner can lead to lots of enjoyable sex, even before you buy anything.

Discuss some of the items and what you would do with them if you owned one. Your partner might be embarrassed to admit that something appeals, but if you get even a hint, indulge yourselves. I've bought lots of toys in my time. Some work; many don't.

But the ones that do are worth all the money you spend on the ones that don't.

Let's take a moment to get specific about toys. There are so many kinds, so let's start with dildos:

- How big should it be? That's a matter of taste and feel, and thickness is much more relevant than length. Big ones seem like a silliness, but remember it's going to go inside her. Will it fit? Probably. A woman's body is made to stretch and accommodate. I wouldn't want anything much larger than Ed. You might want to try a dildo that tapers, narrow at the tip and thicker at the base. That way you can insert it just as far as you like. Some have ridges along the shaft for a different feel. Some are curved to hit the g-spot. I've had several like that and haven't noticed any difference, but I keep trying.

- What should it be made of? There are hard plastic dildos that feel like a rigid erection. They are also very cold when first inserted, and that can be an additional source of excitement. Others are made of softer plastic, ranging eventually to the natural feeling ones made of jellylike plastic.

- Do you want it to look like a real penis or do you want a red, white, and blue rod? Do you care?

- How will you be using it? Do you want to play with a harness? If so, you need a dildo with a wide flange to keep it in place. Do you want one with a suction cup so you can attach it to the edge of the tub and mount it?

- Do you want it for anal play? If so, you need a wide flange to keep it from slipping inside. Remember, the vagina is a closed container, so nothing can get lost. Not so with the anus. A dildo without a flange can be pushed inside and then be difficult and really, really embarrassing to remove.

Next, let's talk about vibrators. There are a few questions you want to answer for yourself and your partner before you buy your first one:

- What do you want to use it for? Is it for insertion or for playing externally? Do you merely want to touch it to your genitals or do you intend to insert it into your vagina or anus? Check chapter 11 for more about anal dildos and vibrators.

- How strong do you want the vibrations to be? If you're using it on your clitoris, less power is needed. Vaginally you might want more. Plug-in models usually have stronger vibrations than those that are battery-operated. If you get one that allows you to vary the speed, you can see what gives the most pleasure. If you purchase a battery-operated one, be sure you have the right-size batteries if they are not included. For the plug-in types, you might want an extension cord for more freedom of movement.

- How much do you want to spend?

- How big do you want it to be? If you're going to keep it at home, size isn't much of an issue. However, if you're going to travel with it, smaller might be more practical. What about the part you insert? All the same issues that we discussed with dildos are relevant for insertable vibrators as well.

- Do you care about its looks? Vibrators come in varied

colors, sizes, and shapes. They come with small projections that buzz on the clitoris while inserted, with beads that move inside for stimulation of your channel, and lots more.

- Can he play too? Of course. A vibrator on the penis or testicles can be dynamite.

In addition to the basics above, there are lots more toys you can buy. Nipple clamps can be enjoyable during games of power and control, or to give a little painful stimulus. A word about clothespins. The ordinary clip-on clothespins that you can buy at the hardware store are too strong for most people who want to play. Those you can buy from toy sites, stores, and catalogs have a weaker pinch.

There are sleeves for him to use on his penis for masturbatory fun. Some vibrate, and most can and should be lubricated. Some look like hands or mouths for added visual stimulation. Some have vacuum devices that create a sucking sensation.

Cock rings are meant to control the blood flowing from his penis so his erection will be harder and last longer. They come in plastic, fabric, rubber, and leather, and can be slid on or fastened around both the penis and testicles. Some men say their orgasms are stronger with one in place; others can't ejaculate until it's removed. If the latter is the case, one that fastens and can be removed quickly is a must.

Lubricants are a necessary part of most toy play, and at other times as well. Use a commercially purchased water-based product, not baby or mineral oil or Vaseline. You need something that's safe in the vagina or anus, and that won't get tacky too quickly. Some lubes are available in your local drugstore, others through catalogs. Try a few to see which works best for you. Oh, and spit doesn't work worth spit (sorry). It stays slippery for about three seconds, then disappears.

Toys

Here's what ordinary folks like you have said about playing with toys in the bedroom (and elsewhere).

How to Give and Get It

A thirty-three-year-old woman wrote:

My husband and I are a very happily married couple who just recently explored the use of sex toys during our lovemaking. This is all new to us, and we both like it a great deal. As any woman knows, oral sex is great, but for me, when you add vaginal stimulation in the form of a dildo, I'm in heaven.

We have tried only a few toys, one being an external vibrator and the other a ten-inch vibrating dildo. Both are wonderful and we enjoy them. Depending on the mood, we will use the vibrator with my husband's tongue to bring me to the perfect orgasm, but at other times when I want to absolutely devour my husband we use the big thing. I am not a big woman, but when I get aroused I go wild and am able to take the whole ten inches in me.

A twenty-eight-year-old woman wrote:

I am a very happily married woman who has a very good sex life. Recently I received a superlarge and superthick dildo from my co-workers for my birthday. I figured that it must be made for someone, although I couldn't imagine who. At the time it was very funny and very outrageous. I showed it to my husband when I got home and we had a good laugh, christening it "The Monster."

My husband and I love to perform oral sex on each other and one night after we had been to a wedding, dancing and drinking, he suggested that we try The Monster out. The thing was very, very big, and I discovered as I held it that it vibrated. I am not that big a woman but I figured what the hell. I knew I could tell him to stop if I didn't like it.

My husband did his magic with his tongue on my clitoris and boobs while I eased the big toy into me. I know that this is not true masturbation, but everyone should try this combination of things. *Wow!* The Monster that I thought was way too big for me fit like a glove and I greatly enjoyed it. After a long session of this, during which I climaxed numerous times, the best was yet to come. My husband stopped, kissed me most passionately, and then entered me and I exploded. That was and will forever be the best of our sessions, maybe even a perfect orgasm.

A forty-one-year-old man wrote:

My wife and I recently ordered something silly from Adam & Eve, a nonpenetrating "butterfly" strap-on vibrator for women. When it arrived we giggled a little at the awkward task of strapping it on, but when it was in place and turned on she went wild. The very intense vibrations jolted her and, as she repositioned it for maximum pleasure, I sucked and played with her breasts. In a short time she was bucking and squirming. I sucked harder while my hands roamed all over. I can't remember her having such an intense orgasm. She came and came and I never let up playing with her breasts and touching her.

We really, really liked that purple butterfly, she feeling it and me watching her go crazy. I was so excited that I couldn't wait for her to remove it (straps and all), so I just lifted it so I could enter her while it was still buzzing. It was a great feeling pumping her wet pussy while the butterfly was humming against my cock. My lover will testify this is designed for ladies, and despite the straps, it is a great sex toy. The ability to turn attention to other spots with the "no hands" feature while the toy is working is a great advantage. They claim it can be worn under clothing . . . we can't wait to try that!

A forty-two-year-old woman wrote:

I didn't think there was any sex toy we hadn't tried, but recently my husband found something on a small Web site that he had to order. He only told me that he had found something new and I couldn't wait to see what it was.

It arrived a few weeks later, on a day we were going to visit some friends for the evening. I have several oversize Mickey Mouse sweatshirts and he suggested that I wear one. I came into the living room and he had put a small box on the coffee table. He told me sit beside him while he opened the package.

Inside were two small sucker-looking things, which he explained were for my nipples. He pulled up my sweatshirt and pulled my bra aside. Using some device on the front, he attached one to each nipple then put my bra back in place. As I pulled down my sweatshirt, I felt a pulling at my nipples but it was so slight that I sort of ignored it.

As the evening progressed the continued sucking on my nipples made them sensitive, and by the time we left to go home I was really hot. Needless to say, I showed him how excited I was in the car when we pulled into the garage.

Never say there's nothing new. There's always something.

A thirty-eight-year-old man wrote:

My thirty-six-year-old wife and I use a soft, pink, eight-inch dildo during perhaps 80 percent of our lovemaking sessions. I can't tell you how much it has enhanced our sex lives. This dildo is two inches longer and quite a bit thicker than I am. At first I worried that my penis wouldn't be enough for her after the dildo but I was completely wrong. When I eventually fuck her she's really satisfied by my equipment. When we play with it inside of her, I actually enjoy thinking of it as another lover. I've never told her that, but I wonder whether she thinks that way too.

A thirty-two-year-old woman wrote:

Toys, toys, toys! Heavens yes. We have dildos of all shapes and sizes, a few in silly colors too. We have a special vibrator just for my husband. He likes different stimulation at different times and it is a fun way to play. The vibrator came with a couple of masturbation sleeves, I guess you'd call them. They're slender tubes that he can insert his cock into and then get a dick massage. His favorite is one of a soft pink jelly material that keeps him company when I am away and joins us in play when the mood strikes. We also have vibrators for me, including my favorite one of waterproof blue jelly. It is close in size to my husband and he likes to join me with it often. We've even played with that one in the shower.

Our favorite toy is one we've learned to enjoy together. It is a soft clear cock ring with an attachment that a vibrating bullet fits into. It provides wonderful stimulation for both of us when we enjoy the woman-on-top position. If a woman ever wanted a perfect orgasm this toy will get her there.

A twenty-seven-year-old man wrote:

I have used metal cock rings and leather cock straps and ball separators. A strap-on with a snap or Velcro is safer, because it can be more easily removed. It is also easier to put on. The one-piece, nonfastening kind that attaches behind the balls is rigid and can only be squeezed into when flaccid. Doing something so blatantly sexually related always starts to arouse me and get me hard so the rigid ring is hard to get on quickly enough.

A tight cock ring and strap is spectacular. It traps blood in the penis, making it much thicker, more rigid, and more sensitive. If sized right, it should make your cock throb, without being painful. It also constricts the testicles a little (a lot with a ball separator), which can cause exciting twinges when they bang into things during sex.

My wife often squeals when I fuck her with a cock ring on. She says it feels like a totally different penis during sex. I don't know that they prevent ejaculation any, but they do reduce the likelihood that I will lose an erection prior to ejaculation.

A forty-nine-year-old man wrote:

Early in our twenty-six-year marriage my wife thought she would never resort to or enjoy toys, but she changed her mind before long. At first we experimented with the simple, cheap plastic bullet-shaped vibrators, and although they got her off, they don't last long.

From there she went to the rabbit-type vibrators—the ones with the separate clit stimulator, rotating shaft, and internal beads. She really liked those, but found they didn't last particularly well either. She also found out she liked penetration with the soft jelly more than the harder latex ones.

About ten years ago she discovered the Eroscillator. This well-made masturbator is no toy. It's a little pricey, about ninety dollars, but it's built for the long haul. Instead of just vibrating, the head oscillates like an electric toothbrush and does it quietly, something my wife likes. The first one we bought is still kicking.

Her favorite technique is to lay it on the right side of her clit, on her favorite sweet spot, and let it do its thing. She likes the Eroscillator so much she said she could sell them door to door. Once she met another woman who owned one, and she loved hers, too. Ladies, my wife encourages you to check one out today.

A forty-two-year-old man wrote:

My wife and I order items from an adult catalog often. Included in our current order was a news-letter, basically stories, info-articles, et cetera. It included an article on Chinese anal love beads and a woman's experience when she brought them

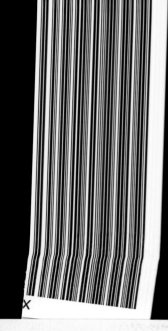

home to her husband, who thoroughly enjoyed the item.

I must mention that we have tried love beads before and, though I enjoyed them, the experience wasn't earth shattering. My mate seemed to appreciate them more. I keep tugging on them lightly while eating her pussy, until I can feel her start to buck, then I start pulling hard enough to pop them out one at a time.

The beads have been in the back of our "love drawer" for a while, but after reading that hot article describing another couple playing with their beads we "pulled them out" (pun intended) of the toy drawer for another go. I'll tell you what, something was just right this time. She pulled them out during my orgasm and I came so hard I thought I would turn inside out. The true benefits of sharing sexual experiences with others.

A fifty-six-year-old man wrote:
My fantasy was always to have my wife do me with a strap-on dildo, just a small one, but I always knew it would be dynamite. Finally, while we were looking at a porn site, I confessed to her. Well, she certainly heard me. Without my knowledge, she ordered one, and we tried it recently. It was the most exciting thing we've ever done, maybe because it's so taboo. Anyway, you asked about the perfect orgasm. I guess I should talk about sharing the climax with my wife, but when I climaxed with her hand on me and that dildo fucking me from behind—it was the most perfect one I can ever remember.

A sixty-eight-year-old man wrote:

One of my greatest desires is to have my wonderful wife of almost forty years take me with a strap-on. I have absolutely no interest in having another man fuck me, but I nearly melt at the thought of having my wife strap on a large member and bend me over for some serious strokes while she pleasures herself at the same time with another vibrator. I'm hard at the mere thought. Maybe I'll buy one and give it to her as a present. For me!

A fifty-one-year-old woman wrote:

Ben wa balls with strings attached really work. When you place them in your vagina and rock back and forth with your knees up, you can feel a slight stimulation. I like walking around the house wearing them, for up to fifteen minutes because they also strengthen the PC muscle like doing Kegel exercises. Basically the longer you wear them the stronger that muscle becomes, and the stronger the PC muscle, the more you can squeeze your guy during sex. Sometimes, while we're on a long car trip, I tell my husband that I'm wearing them. It keeps us both thinking of what we'll do when we reach our destination.

Here's a hint. Tug on the string as if you're trying to pull them out but squeeze and try to keep them in. It feels great and strengthens those muscles still more. I've even had my husband try to pull them out as I try to keep them in. Boy, it excites us both and leads to many great climaxes.

Kegel Exercises

And speaking of Kegel exercises . . . As we women age, the muscles that clench during orgasm become weaker. Those are the same ones, by the way, that help with bladder control. Kegel exercises are easy to do and you can, as the writer of the previous letter points out, tighten those muscles with delicious results.

How to Get It for Her

To do Kegels, begin by sitting on the toilet and urinating. Try to stop the stream in the middle by tightening the necessary muscles, just to let your brain know which ones they are. Eventually you'll be able to isolate those muscles and clench them at will. Now do so. Often. Quickly clench and release, then hold them tightly for several minutes. Increase the speed of clench and release, and the length of clenches. Keep doing Kegels and you'll find that both you and your lover will realize the difference.

A forty-three-year-old man wrote:

> My girlfriend has learned to control her vaginal muscles and this has resulted in wonderful new sex for us. The Kegel muscles that she uses to stop peeing can be used to stimulate the penis during intercourse. We like to use the position of her on her back with her legs spread, knees bent, and feet up in the air. This tilts her vagina up, and is a good position for thrusting.
>
> After she guides my penis into her vagina and thrusting starts, her vagina muscles grip my penis as it pushes inside her. As I pull the penis back in preparation for another thrust, her vagina relaxes,

and I can feel the gripping and relaxing of her vagina on the shaft of my penis. Sometimes I just push my penis inside her and she stimulates it by gripping and relaxing her muscles.

This tight grip during thrusting also stimulates her because of the gentle tugging on the hood of her clitoris. We also use the doggy-style that lets me play with her breasts and nipples during thrusting, and I can also reach around and rub her clitoris. When I ejaculate, I stop the thrusting and I love the feeling of her vagina sort of "milking" the last few drops of semen from my penis.

Chapter 9

TALKING DIRTY, PHONE SEX, AND ROLE PLAYING

TALKING DIRTY ISN'T EXACTLY WHAT YOU THINK.
Yes, it can be really arousing to use those hot four-letter words during lovemaking, or before, as great foreplay. "I'm going to stick my cock into you later until you scream," or "Fuck me harder," or "I love sucking your tits," or "What a sweet pussy you have," can really ignite the passion of both lovers. However, that's not necessarily the best place to start.

How to Give It

Let's say you want to see what happens when you whisper sweet somethings into your lover's ear. Begin with words that are just a bit more risqué than the ones you usually use. If you're really proper, start with "I love making love with you" at a strategic moment. Or "Oh baby, you feel so good." Or something really simple, like, "Do it, do it, do it." Just breaking the silence in the bedroom can be a great beginning to dirty talking. From there you can branch out in whatever direction you like. Oh, and if it makes you a little uncomfortable, that's fine. The slight edge of embarrassment can be exciting in itself.

How to Get It

Suppose you've always wanted your partner to talk dirty to you before or during lovemaking. Well, if you do it, gently at first, he or she might be encouraged to do the same. If you want to go a bit farther, here's a delicious idea.

A *twenty-seven-year-old woman* wrote:

> I was always really proper. I like that word better than *prudish*. I never said *shit* or like that. When my husband and I married we had a good sex life but I sensed that he wanted to go a bit farther. From time to time he asked me to talk a little dirty in bed, but I just couldn't. It frustrated him, but it frustrated me even more. I wanted to do it for him, but no way.
>
> One evening we were petting on the couch and he began to touch me between my legs. It made me so hungry. He kept stroking and rubbing until I thought I would climax right there but we got up, undressed, and climbed into bed. To my surprise, he lay on his side of the bed and didn't touch me. Then he whispered, "Do you want me?"
>
> "God, yes," I said.
>
> "Tell me."
>
> "I want you. I really do."
>
> "Tell me exactly what you want."

After a few stutters, I said, "I want you to touch me like you were doing before. Then make love to me." For that night it was enough, but I now know that he was building me up to bigger and better things.

A few nights later he was pinching my nipples the way I like and he said, "What do you want me to do now?" I was totally tongue-tied. "Tell me or I won't do anything." When I kept silent, he said, "Say, *I want you to play with my tits. Say tits.*" I just couldn't, but he kept me so excited that I finally gave in. I whispered that one word, and that was all he needed.

Well, it kept on like that for a long time and I got more and more used to using those words in bed. I still can't use them in public, of course, and I'm a bit twitchy just writing to you, but my husband is sitting beside me, playing with my pussy (he told me to write that).

A forty-one-year-old woman wrote:

A while ago, my boyfriend introduced me to telling stories in the dark. We lie beside each other, sometimes fully dressed, and one of us begins an erotic story. In the beginning we just used our imaginations but now I hunt the Net for great starters. The one who begins sets the scene, the characters, and what's happening, then turns the story over to the other for the next act. Back and forth it goes, wandering into things we wouldn't really do but are such fun to imagine: threesomes, orgies, doing it in a taxi with the driver watching. We've done it, in our minds at least, everywhere and in every way imaginable. We've even gotten into rape fantasies, which excite me more than I can ever say.

I know we'd never actually do any of the things we fantasize about, but the dreams are better anyway, more perfect and less threatening.

A fifty-year-old man wrote:

I remember my first experience with talking dirty very well. I'm a landscaper, and I was feeling completely exhausted from all the physical exercise I had been doing over the previous few days at work. To make matters worse it had been really sunny and the heat had made me feel even more exhausted. I was in bed with my girlfriend and struggling to get as hard as I usually do. I was erect but just not rock hard.

Then something happened. For the first time ever a woman started talking dirty to me. She began cautiously by telling me how wet I made her as she gripped and pumped my cock in her soft hand. Was I dreaming? I replied by saying that I loved what she was doing to me and how it felt soooo good. She must have felt me get harder instantly as I became incredibly turned on. This encouraged her further.

She talked about how hot she was and how hot I made her. Then she focused more on how big and hard I was, how good I felt in her hand, and how she wanted to feel me sliding into her dripping wet body. No really dirty words, just incredibly erotic ideas. It was wonderful for a tired working guy. I guess she knew quite well what she was doing to me so she just kept going.

During all this she would look down to see the tip of my cock pushing in and out from between her hand too. All this talk and increased pumping had the desired result and I started heavy breathing and thrust my hips forward in ecstacy. I finally came in hard spasms.

That was probably one of the most perfect orgasms and erotic experiences ever. It took me a few minutes to recover and come back down to earth. Then, a little later, I fucked her brains out having no trouble getting hard as steel.

Unfortunately we split up soon after but I would dearly love to repeat that amazing experience with another woman. The brain is the best sex organ, you just need to stimulate it. I get really hard every time I think about it (including now).

A fifty-seven-year-old man wrote:
My wife of thirty years really knows how to get to me. Often, when we're out of the house, at a restaurant, play, or party, she'll whisper something dirty into my ear. Sometimes she'll say, "Is your big, hard cock hot for me tonight?" Or she might whisper, "My pussy's all wet. Just wait until later and you can suck on my tits."

Hearing my neatly dressed, proper little wife saying really naughty things never ceases to get me really turned on. Fast!

Phone Sex

Phone sex can be used to excite a faraway lover or heat things up in a situation where neither partner can do anything about it. It arouses both the giver and the receiver. One writer wrote that she and her husband have two phone lines and they actually phone each other from different rooms of the house to play and tease.

Why would you play with phone sex either with a distant lover or with someone who's right there with you? I think the answer is obvious. It's fun, and increases the anticipation of the next time you're going to be together.

How to Give and Get It

Phone your lover at work, especially if he or she doesn't have a private office. If you begin a little dirty talking in a situation in which your partner can't reply, it can be fabulously frustrating. Sometimes it's difficult to know how to begin. Try:

- "Hi, honey. I was just remembering last night. Do you know what felt best?" Then describe it in elaborate detail.

- "I was wondering whether you're coming home early. If you do, I'll be wearing . . ."

- "I can't wait until we're alone. I was reading a story about . . ."

- Or you can get right to it. "I'm thinking about your sweet pussy and how good it will feel to slide my dick into it."

You can even go so far as to masturbate while you're on the phone, telling your partner every move you're making.

A thirty-one-year-old woman wrote:

> My fiancé and I met long distance. The phone and letters were all that we had. Before we had even been intimate with each other in person, erotic letters and phone sex came into play. These were both very new things for me. It took a little while to be able to verbalize on the phone what I wanted to do to him and what I wanted him to do to me—but, oh, did he drive me crazy telling me what he wanted to do to me! After about a month of this, all kinds of things started coming out of my mouth. And the orgasms on both ends were explosive, to say the least.
>
> I found that it was easier for me to open up and talk dirty to him by starting out with "I had this dream about us last night . . ." Somehow it was just easier and made it a little less threatening for me. And I haven't stopped since.

A fifty-two-year-old man wrote:

> I used to have phone sex frequently with my first wife when we were apart. I broached the topic the first time by reliving a typical sexual experience and we wandered down memory lane discussing an evening we particularly remembered. While we were talking I quietly mentioned that I'd removed my slacks and was playing with myself. I told her in detail exactly what I was doing and she returned the favor. It was the most erotic thing to hear how excited she was getting. She was breathing so hard that soon it got difficult for her to talk.

Eventually she climaxed and then I stroked myself and came too.

From then on we'd do it often. Unfortunately I can't get my new wife interested, but I'm still trying.

A thirty-one-year-old man wrote:

My first year out of college, my now-wife was still a senior, and my job took me halfway across the country. We could only see one another about once every two months. Given the circumstances, playing on the phone was the best we could do, and I'd recommend it to any couple that has to be apart more than a few days at a time.

I've never been turned on by the thought of having phone sex with a stranger, though, and for that reason I would never consider patronizing a commercial phone sex operation. Phone sex for me was a strategy for staying intimately in touch with my partner rather than being turned on by some stranger. The fact that it was my then-girlfriend made it particularly special.

A forty-one-year-old woman wrote:

I am in a relationship with a sweet, loving man also in his forties whose business causes him to travel much of the time. Since I also work, I can't go along so we do what we can online and by phone.

For our first time, I bought a vibrator to play with. We both lie in bed hundreds of miles apart, describing everything for the other . . . lighting, position, music, et cetera. I told him what I would

like to be doing to him and he told me exactly how
and where to use the vibrator.

Now we do this a lot. I have quite a collection
of toys and he tells me exactly what to use and
how to use it. It's very erotic, and my orgasms are
pretty intense while using a dildo or vibrator and
hearing his soft, sensuous voice in my ear.
Somehow, the use of a toy seems to make our
time together on the phone much more intimate.
We love it.

Role Playing

On the road to building the perfect orgasm, you might enjoy a night
of role playing. I know that to some of you this sounds silly—
costumes and stories, pretending to be someone else—and if it isn't
your thing, as I've said over and over in this book, forget it. But if you
think that climbing out of your persona to take on someone else's
might lead to a freedom you don't otherwise have, then this might be
the section for you.

Like what? Let's see what some real people have to say about
role playing.

How to Give It

A twenty-six-year-old woman wrote:

My boyfriend and I have been together for about a
year. Our sex life is absolutely the best but he asked
me recently what we could do to spice it up even a
little more—you know, just so we won't get bored

doing the same ol' same ol'. When I didn't know how to answer he brought up role playing. So far we've only thought up about three things that we could role-play:

1. We could act like we don't know each other, and just want to have a one-night stand and have sex.

2. After dinner out at a restaurant he could go get the car while I wait outside looking like I need a ride. He could come along and ask whether I need a lift and I'd reluctantly agree. I'd jump into his car acting as if I don't know him but I'd obviously be turned on by him. I could start to give him oral sex that would eventually turn into more erotic stuff once we got home.

3. My boyfriend came up with this one. We could get a hotel room and then he could knock on the door looking for someone else. I could lure him inside and seduce him.

Of course there are more to these stories; that's just the brief version.

And a fifty-three-year-old man wrote:
Role playing? God, yes! We've enjoyed that for many years, and this year makes thirty-two happy, sexy years together.
Some of our favorite roles are:

1. Dancer and the peep-show customer.

2.   High-class escort and client.

3.   Beginner escort and client.

Can someone loosen up and let themselves go? Of course! That's the beauty of role playing. If a person can recapture the childhood delight of playing make-believe and get into a particular character, the possibilities are endless. You can indulge as much of your fantasy as you desire. You don't have to know anything about acting; just imagine it's Halloween and go with the character. It's your own little sexual mini play; enjoy!

Here's a way to get into role playing without having to actually do anything.

A forty-six-year-old man wrote:

We haven't made it to the point where we do real costume-type role playing (the French Maid outfit, the School Girl Uniform, et cetera) . . . yet. A good alternative for my wife and me has been to remember that piece of advice from many who counsel folks on sexual relationships—your brain is your biggest sex organ.

What I have become quite comfortable doing, during lovemaking, is to tell my wife to keep her eyes closed and imagine. "Imagine you are the naughty schoolgirl bent over my office desk with your panties down around your ankles and about to be caned." Or, "Imagine you are the mistress of a powerful Roman emperor, brought into the main hall where hundreds are about to witness your obedience as you are stripped naked and made to service every desire of a dozen sex-deprived soldiers just returned from battle." And so it goes. The sky's the limit isn't it?

Whereas many scenarios might seem silly if acted out, my experience has been that my panting spouse thoroughly enjoys the trips our brain has taken us on. Give it a try.

How to Get It

There are many ways to begin, and the previous letter is a good example of one. Telling stories in the dark during sex is a great way to climb into another personality without the risk of getting dressed up and actually playing a part. Think of a scene that might curl your toes—and your partner's, of course. Then just tell the story.

Not only can this lead to a hot situation, but it will also give you lots of information about what your partner's tastes are. He or she might reveal something long hidden but delicious:

- "You've got an appointment with the doctor for a checkup. You arrive and go into the little exam room, remove all your clothes, and get ready." Then you can toss the story to your partner. "What do you think might happen when the doctor comes in?"

- "We're snowed in at a small ski hut in the mountains. All the roads are blocked and it looks like we're going to be here for a while. I prowl around and find that there's plenty of food, a bottle of very good Cabernet, and lots of wood for the fire. What do you think you'll do while I build a fire?"

- "I'm a prostitute and you're the customer. You've hired

me for the evening and I'm going to give you your
money's worth. Where should I begin?"

During the storytelling, you can take your time describing
what you both are wearing, what the room looks like—all the
details that will slow down the action, making the anticipation
build and giving you both time to consider how far you want
the story, and your subsequent lovemaking, to go.

We'll get into power fantasies later in this book, but this
might be a good way to explore those too:

- "I've failed my math exam and I'm desperate to keep this
  news from my parents. You're my teacher and I'll do anything if you just won't tell them."

- "I'm the guard who locks down your prison cell each
  night. After lights-out I come back, open your cell, and
  walk inside. You don't dare say anything since I've got all
  the power."

- "I've got a magic ring that, when you look into the stone,
  puts you under my spell. I wonder what I'll have you do
  first."

I think you've gotten the idea. Once you've played in your imag-
ination for a while, you can branch out into actually acting out a scenario if you wish. Play doctor and patient or masseuse and customer.
Try stripper and voyeur or older, knowledgeable neighbor and
teenager. There are so many possibilities that I'm sure you have
something in mind even now.

Here's a letter from a thirty-eight-year-old man in the UK who
actually acted out one of his most delightful fantasies:

Dear Joan,

I thought you'd be interested in this story. I had a girlfriend who loved role playing and had some very cheeky, sexy ideas about it. She'd read a book on schools in the UK in which punishment sessions were described and, knowing that I'd been to such a school, wanted to know more. In fact, this punishment had stopped years before my time, but she still went on and on about it. So I had an idea: Why not role play?

Now, I should say that I don't think role playing is something for beginners, and that it only works if each partner knows the other well and, most importantly, appreciates his or her limits. If someone says no, then that's it. But if you can really trust one another, and keep everything under control, it can be wonderful and stretch you and your lover's imaginations. I think you'll see what I mean!

Anyway, I discussed the idea of playing professor and student with this adventurous lady and she readily agreed. Of course, she knew that I wouldn't hurt her, but the thought of a new experience certainly excited her.

"Can we do it now?" she asked.

"Of course not," I replied. "You haven't done anything wrong yet."

To cut a long story short, my bedroom was reassigned as the professor's study, and she needed help with her schoolwork. She knocked on the

door and came in, wearing a short skirt and cling-
ing T-shirt. "Please sir, I can't do these physics
problems. Could you help me?"

"Yes, of course, Miss Smith. I'd be pleased to.
Do sit here." At this point my acting abilities rather
failed me, but the general idea was that I tried to
explain some detail or other to her, while she sat
close to me.

She was a bit more eager than I was so she
said, "Thank you sir, I understand now. Gosh, it's
hot in here; do you mind if I take my T-shirt off
before we do the next question?"

"You certainly may not. You're not allowed to
strip in school. Please wait until you get home. Miss
Smith, I told you not to do that. Put it on again," I
said to the bare-chested girl in a stern voice.

"Sorry sir. Will I be punished?"

"Yes you will be. I'll have to check in the rules
to see what it will be."

"I do hope it won't be the slipper, sir!" she said,
an adorable little hitch in her voice.

I tried not to smile at the delectable little thing
she'd become. "Yes, I'm afraid it will be. It says
here in the rules that you are to get six strokes."

"Is that on my hand sir?"

"No, you are to bend over a chair!" I tried to
sound stern but it was difficult not to grin as the
scene played out. And my cock was already really
hard.

"Oh sir, I'm terribly sorry. Please don't do that."

"I'm afraid it has to be done for your own good." So the unfortunate girl's fate was decided. I drew up a chair. "Lean over with your hands on the seat, and hold up your skirt," I ordered.

"But sir, I don't think I can do both at the same time."

"Right. You'll have to take your skirt off then." Thus revealed were the most delicious, frilly knickers with cutaway sides and back, showing, as she went over the chair, the full loveliness of her slim shape. "I've decided to reduce the punishment by using my hand instead of the slipper," I announced.

"Thank you sir." This was just an excuse to stroke her with my palm and run it over her panties. Once or twice, my hand just happened to catch the lace and pull everything to the side. At each sensuous touch, she wriggled slightly and moved her feet farther apart, showing even more to me.

"Now get up," I commanded after I'd administered her six swats.

"Oh sir, that really hurt me," she said, rubbing the affected area with one hand so that the front of the panties came down.

"It should have taught you a good lesson," I said. Whereupon she gave me a lesson, the theme of which was passionate lovemaking with a tigress.

The "return" match at her flat was, as I expected, even more playful. I became the student and she the school's headmistress. This time the rules stated that I had to be fully stripped. She was hardly able to conceal her delight at the prospect of my bare flesh. Instead of using a slipper, she had a soft brush, and subjected me to the most excruciating tickling. My embarrassment at the uncontrollable dribbling from my cock caused her great amusement.

I've played such games with a few girlfriends since, which has always lead to fabulous lovemaking.

If this sort of thing sounds like fun, go for it. It's hot and can lead to some perfect orgasms. I should know. Ed and I have tried quite a few.

Chapter 10

KICK IT UP A NOTCH

Water—A New Sex Toy

Water as a sex toy? You bet. Did you know there are dildos that can be filled with warm or cold water to give an extra thrill? But here, we're talking about good old faucet water. Making love in the shower, hot tub, or pool can add a delicious bit of spice to your sex life. And it solves a few problems related to hygiene too. Feeling really clean can encourage oral sex, and water trickling, flowing, or pounding over lovers' bodies feels delicious. Don't overlook the masturbatory possibilities either.

How to Get It

A forty-six-year-old man wrote:
> Masturbating in the shower is the best. It's truly private and I can play to my heart's content. I love my shower massager too. I have a handheld one

that gets to those places you can't see. There is nothing like doing an inventory on your assets and having the shower massager stimulating your scrotum. I can let it pound against my asshole. That's a sensation that always makes me lose it quickly.

I love to bring my playmates in the bath and just fool around. I don't know why being in warm water seems to lessen inhibitions, but it does. And, of course, we can play with oral sex without worrying about smells and stuff.

Never had so much dirty fun getting clean.

A thirty-five-year-old woman wrote:

I love to masturbate in the shower and tub. I remember being in the fifth grade taking baths and enjoying playing with the jets of water from the handheld shower. Little did I know then that I was having orgasms. Since I learned what an orgasm was, my sex life has always been fulfilling. I've learned to take charge of my sexuality and ensure that I always am satisfied. I most enjoy playing in a Jacuzzi with my man. Those jets of water hitting various spots on my body are electrifying.

My husband gave me a handheld shower massager especially for when I'm away from home, and I use it a lot. I travel often for business and, when I have a phone in the bathroom of my hotel, I call him and tell him how naughty I'm being. It's heaven.

How to Give It

A fifty-eight-year-old man wrote:

Married for just over thirty-one years, my wife and I decided to remodel our bathroom and make the shower stall large enough for two people. My wife loves as hot a shower as humanly possible, but after washing we turn the temperature down and let the slightly cooler water tantalize her breasts and nipples.

While standing behind her, I add both hands to this thrilling adventure. When her front is thoroughly taken care of she turns to face me with the streams of water running down the crease in her very round backside. With my hands and cock providing any extras she desires, we have found the streams hitting strategic body parts can be a very exciting addition to our showers. It might not be for everybody, but it sure brightens up our days.

Showers aren't just for getting clean. How about getting dirty! Invite your lover to climb in with you one evening when you've got time to play. Use lots of lather and take time to clean *everywhere*. Buy new soap with a different scent. Fill the bathroom with candles, taking care to keep them away from any paper products. Get one of those European hose showers and play.

Last year Ed and I installed a fancy showerhead with a misting setting. On hot summer nights we open the bathroom window to let in the scents and sounds of the outdoors and play in the soft mist.

Baths are really adult playpens. Use lots of bubbles and soapy hands. Rub and stroke with everything from soft sponges and cloths to rough, scratchy loofahs. Wash each other's hair, a very sexy activity. Oh, and if your tub isn't big enough for two, finding a way to share can lead to lots of tangled legs, arms, and other parts. Ain't tangling fun?

Don't overlook the possibility of skinny-dipping or romping in the hot tub. Ever tried sitting your partner on the kitchen counter and playing with the veggie sprayer? Water is everywhere, and always fun to play with. Look for possibilities.

Watching Sexy Movies

I've read that women aren't as turned on by visual erotica as men are, but from a personal viewpoint I have to disagree. I've been with many men and had long-term relationships with several. None of them was ever turned on by X-rated films. However, I am. I like ones with a real plot, but I get really turned on by watching couples make love. The participants have to look like they are enjoying it, despite cameras, lighting, and such, of course. In addition, I sometimes find techniques I can add to my repertoire.

Let's see what others have to say about watching erotic films.

How to Get It

A thirty-five-year-old man wrote:
My wife and I recently got a satellite dish and subscribe to two triple-X-rated channels. Now we have hot porn twenty-four hours a day, seven days a week. The cost is about $120 a year and it's very well worth it.

Most of the movies have some minor plot, but

basically they're about sex, sex, sex! I guess they are really poor, but who cares. They make great fore-play. I prefer the visual part and I recently found out my wife likes the audio. She closes her eyes and listens while I "play" on her body.

A forty-seven-year-old man wrote:

Big *grin*. I rented an X-rated film a few years ago and mentioned to my wife that I'd like to watch it with her. Her first reaction was, "Why do you need to watch 'that'? Isn't what we do enough?" It slowly evolved into, "If you insist."

So we watched together in bed, holding hands. At first she was quick to remark on which women had had breast implants or tummy tucks. "Boy, does that look phony." Slowly, however, she got turned on. That night's sex was terrific. Now I rent a film once a month or so. She still insists it's not her thing, but I know differently.

A twenty-eight-year-old woman wrote:

I know that most women are turned off by porno flicks, but I have a different view on the subject. I love watching them with my boyfriend, and don't have any problem with it. I like especially watching men with large penises (and my boyfriend gets turned on too).

It's difficult to rent them in my town, but there's a theater where you can go to watch. We pay for a private booth and sit down to watch the movie. I love any movie with loads of oral sex and come shots.

We both get turned on by the pretty girls with cocks in their mouths too, and I always treat

my boyfriend with a good blow job. Well, that's
my confession, and no one who knows me
would guess—except my sexy boyfriend. Come
on girls, stop the automatic "I'm not interested"
and get into it. You'd be amazed what a turn-on it
might be.

Okay, I know it's embarrassing to go into a video store and rent
an X-rated film. "Everyone there will know . . ." They probably won't
care, and if they notice, let them wonder what delicious things you
and your partner are going to do tonight.

Movies can be so *expanding*. The characters might do something really arousing that neither of you had thought of, or that you
never had the nerve to mention. A comment like "Gee, that looks
interesting" might spark a period of communication that can lead
to totally new activities or just variations on familiar themes.

Many people just like to watch people making love, and if that's
what turns you on, great. Others, however, want some kind of a
story, and it can be really difficult to find adult films that have a plot.
If you want one with more than cum shots, I've found that videos by
Femme Productions seem to have good story lines blended with
great sex. You might have to rent quite a few to find one that turns
you both on. Don't hesitate to turn off any you don't like and begin
a new one. As the saying goes, "You have to kiss a lot of frogs to find
one handsome prince."

During the film it can be fun to see how long you two can
watch without touching. If you have a film with lots of different
activities, try using the FAST FORWARD button for a random length of
time, then agree to do whatever the characters are doing when you
press *play*.

Making Erotic Films

Erotic movies used to be almost impossible for amateurs to make at home, but in the age of video recorders it's a cinch. Set up a camera and just let it roll. You might want to begin slowly, with a scene of one person undressing, to become used to the idea of the camera. Then you can graduate to photographing each other's genitals and masturbation. Finally, you can set the camera on the dresser or on a tripod (if you have one) and have a blast.

How to Get It

A forty-year-old woman wrote:

My husband and I bought a video camera recently and decided to make home porn. We read through the owner's manual to look for any features to use for our video and we discovered that our camera was equipped with night vision capability. Night vision allows you to record tape in complete darkness by using infrared light. The only problem is everything recorded appears green. The nice thing about the night vision is that I am one of the many women who is self-conscious about my body. I thought that being in the dark would make me more comfortable with being videotaped completely naked.

We set the camera up on a tripod, turned off all the lights, kissed, gave each other oral sex, and continued with the best sex we've had in a long time. It made me feel great to be able to please my husband this way, and know that we can watch the tape afterward, anytime we want.

Now I know you're probably asking, "Who wants to watch porn when everything is green?" Well let me tell you, you don't see all the flaws with your body. I still had my fat, but no stretch marks, cellulite, or scars. I really felt beautiful that night, and I am slowly getting more comfortable with the camera. It was a great new experience for us.

A *thirty-one-year-old woman wrote:*

We never really set out to video ourselves making love but my husband, Tom, accidentally (on purpose?) left the recorder going one day while we had sex. We watched it later and I was less mortified than I thought I'd be. Despite my initial reluctance to see myself in all my naked glory (?) I got totally turned on, as did Tom. We fucked for hours.

As we watched again we realized that the result was pretty poor and as we talked about how turned on we had become, we decided to go for it and record a proper scene. We went out and bought a new camera with a handheld control, and set about making our own porn movie.

Perhaps the films we've made are not up to professional standards but we enjoy our little fantasies and find it all a big turn-on—both making and watching the videos. We have thought about getting someone in to record us but are not sure about how to go about it. From our experience we can honestly say most people enjoy looking at themselves on video, and recording yourselves making love is no different.

Watching the film later can be as much of a turn-on as making it was. Find a time when you can play while you see yourself making love on the screen. It might take a few minutes to get past the sight of yourself and the embarrassment, but it's worth it. It's like the best of all the worlds—a porno flick with you and your partner as the stars.

Playing Erotic Games

Playing erotic games might seem silly, but sometimes it's great to be silly. Laughter is as much a part of the perfect orgasm as arousal, so relax and see whether some of these ideas appeal to you.

A forty-one-year-old man wrote:

My wife and I discovered many years ago that games can be fun and can help keep the boredom away in a long-term relationship such as ours. So we played a few, trading ideas for ways to pick places, positions, and such. A few years back I noticed that the Post-it note company makes blue and pink pads as well as the standard yellow. That inspired me to create a new erotic game.

I bought pads of the pink and blue stick-on note pages, then got an empty cube-type tissue box. I asked my wife to write down all of her wildest sexual desires and fantasies on the pink notes, fold them, and drop them in the empty tissue box. I did the same on the blue notes. It took a while for us to get "down and dirty" but eventually there were a large number of little folded papers in the box. Ever since, whenever some wild thought hits one of us, we write it down and add our blue and pink notes in the box.

Now the game. Every few weeks, when we're feeling adventurous, we each draw a note of the right color. She reads the request on the blue slip and I read the pink. We then comply with the other's wishes. Of course we each retain veto power in case something just isn't going to work, and each of us has used that to request the draw of another slip.

I have requested that she strip and dance naked for me. She has asked that I perform solo for her viewing pleasure. We have both suggested a quickie outside when the neighbors were partying on their deck just a few feet away. She has suggested that I watch her do a solo, and that I do the same and come on her bosom.

One of the wildest was the night our game resulted in mutual oral pleasure in a big Chicago high-rise hotel within view of office workers in neighboring buildings. The game can be fun and I share it with you for the joy of it all.

A sixty-one-year-old man wrote:
Remember Madonna's Truth or Dare? Well, it's particularly delicious when my wife and I play it. Since we've been married for more than thirty years it's difficult to find a truth that we don't already know, but neither of us has asked for "truth" in quite a long time. Why should we, when the dares are so much fun?

Our dares have ended up with us making love in a cemetery at two in the morning, on the diving board at our condo's pool in the middle of the night, and on our deck while people sit within listening range. We've spent quite a bit of time without undies in various situations. Recently my wife spent an evening at the movies with a dildo held inside her by her panties, and a few weeks ago I wore a cock ring for most of a day at work.

Once you get over the embarrassment, dares can be such a fabulous way to get to do all the really creative things they write about in stories on the Net. Actually, that's where I get some of my ideas. One evening I had her read a particularly raunchy story out loud and on another she printed a picture of a girl in full bondage from a Web site and made me spend half an hour with my hand loosely on my cock, describing the picture.

Now that we're into it we've gotten so many ideas we'll never run out.

A thirty-eight-year-old woman wrote:
I never thought I'd get interested in bedroom games. Sex for me was wonderful, but quite straight. When I met my now-husband ten years ago, he was much more open and light about sex. It was difficult for me to loosen up so he suggested we play a variation on the old game called statues.

We set an oven timer for ten minutes, and *it* would have to get into whatever position the other said. Then *it* couldn't move, no matter what, until the timer went off.

The first few times each of us tried to make the other laugh or move. Sometimes we would succeed and the loser had to do the dishes or something. Finally I decided I to take advantage of the situation. One evening I laid him out on the bed and took my ten minutes to explore his body through his clothes in a way I had never been brave enough to do before.

The next time he was *it* I asked him to wear an old pair of sweats and I again laid him on the bed. I must admit that that evening I cheated and set the timer for twenty minutes. Then I slowly cut his clothes off and played with him. The only part of him that moved was his cock, as it got bigger and bigger. I watched it and discovered what made it twitch and grow. It was quite a learning experience.

Now we occasionally play the same game, naked, with the collection of sex toys we've bought since I got brave. Oh, and I learned that he had hoped that the game would end up where it did. He just gave me time to make it happen.

A fifty-nine-year-old man wrote:

If sex is adult recreation, as experts claim, then "games" can add spice. I'm writing about two such games that my wife and I played long ago. It all began in 1968 during military service while stationed in a major U.S. city. We played a variation on the old childhood game spin-the-bottle.

This spin the bottle variation involved four adult couples all in their early twenties. Those were the wide-open, free-loving 1960s, and sex was pretty free in our community. Not swapping, mind you, just lots of playing in public. This game was obviously preplanned as part of a party held in one couple's apartment. All invitees were told to wear casual clothing. Women were told to wear loose skirts with sweaters and no bras. Men were instructed to wear jeans and sweatshirts only.

When the game began, all couples were seated in a circle, men and women alternating. A soft drink bottle was used as the spinner/pointer. If the neck pointed to a woman, she had the option of exposing her breasts or her genital area for fifteen seconds for all to gaze at and comment upon—nice remarks, of course. If it pointed to a man he had to expose his genitals for the same type of discussion. If the bottle pointed to a woman for a second time, she had no options. If she exposed her breasts on round one, she had to flash her femininity on the second round. The game continued until everyone had been "it" for two rounds. There was no touching during the game.

After the game, needless to say, we were all hot as firecrackers. Someone suggested that we all have sex in the same room, but that idea was quickly vetoed. We were open about our bodies but not interested in the amount of voyeurism that might result. Instead we all disappeared to different rooms for a bit of privacy. My girlfriend and I ended up in the den and I think I had what might have been a nearly perfect orgasm. I guess the only drawback was that it was fast.

Several months later, another couple devised the second game, called Spotlight. The same group assembled, naked, in totally dark room. One half of a couple shined a flashlight on the exposed genitals of the other while commenting on their beauty and the excitement that their body generates. The exposed player can touch and stroke for the enjoyment of the watchers. Like the spin-the-bottle game, everyone gets a turn at being voyeur and exhibitionist. The important part is that the light is never to be on the exposed player's face. Only pussies and dicks are in the spotlight, exposed and played with while others watch under the cover of darkness.

I have never encountered anything like either of those games again, but I have thought about them over the years. The memories never fail to bring a grin to my face.

As you've seen, variations on kids' games can be fun for adults. Remember statues? One of you can get into a position and try to remain completely still while the other partner tries to break that concentration. You can set the rules—no touching or lots of touching, for instance, above and/or below the belt.

There is body paint available to let each of you decorate the other's naked body using fingers or, for a different feel, brushes. A purple penis? Green nipples? Most paints are merely soap that washes off in the shower. Which is more fun, the painting or washing? I'll leave that up to you.

SIDE DISHES

Chapter 11

ANAL SEX

ANAL SEX IS A VOLATILE TOPIC, AND IF YOU'RE sure it isn't your thing, then, as always, I suggest that you skip this chapter. But think twice before reacting with a knee-jerk "I just couldn't." You never know what might curl your toes, or your partner's.

Why are people interested in anal sex? Lots of reasons. First, it's taboo, and forbidden fruit always seems sweeter. Second, lots of the nerves that surround the genitals also travel around the anus. In addition, for a man, a woman's anus will probably be a tighter fit than the vagina and thus more arousing.

Let's get one thing straight. Anal sex isn't just anal intercourse. Sometimes just touching the anal area during foreplay can ignite your partner's passion. There are a few things we have to talk about before we get to letters from real folks who enjoy anal sex in one form or another.

The most basic thing you need to discover is whether your partner is interested. Of course you can come right out and ask. You might learn a lot; he might be eager to experiment, or not the slightest bit interested or curious. Abide by your partner's wishes if he doesn't want to play. But be sure that you're getting an honest answer, and not just what your lover thinks he should say. If you think there's a chance you're not getting the straightest answer, discuss it at more length. Elaborate on your desires and you might be surprised at the end result (sorry, I couldn't resist the pun).

Warning: Anal intercourse is a *high-risk* activity. Lots of diseases are transmitted via fluid-to-blood contact, and during anal intercourse, membranes are usually slightly torn, allowing semen to come in contact with blood. These slight tears don't necessarily result in real injury, but a slight abrasion opens the skin barrier to any deadly viruses that might lurk in semen. I don't care if your lover swears on a stack of Bibles ten feet high that you're the only one he or she has ever been with, don't play without a condom (better still, two condoms). No guessing or taking anyone's word for it. This is a life-and-death decision.

Many couples use condoms for cleanliness' sake as well. Sex in general is a messy business, and anal sex is messier than vaginal intercourse. So let's agree that you should use a condom anyway. Condoms also facilitate switching from anal to vaginal play. Removing a condom eliminates most of the risk of cross-contamination.

Understand that the anal area is full of very dangerous bacteria that would just love a warm, damp home—say, in a vaginal canal or a urethra. Never, and I mean never, touch a woman's vagina after your fingers have been in contact with her anus—not only inside but anywhere in the neighborhood. Use the other hand for stroking or wash your hands well with lots of antibacterial soap. Here's a tip. If you're going to play anally, use a rubber glove or, if you want to be more subtle, slip a condom over your finger. That way you can remove it before any vaginal play and not have to jump up and head for the bathroom.

If you're going to do more than just play outside the rectum, use lots of water-based lubricant. You can get several different kinds at stores, or shop on the Net. As I've said before, petroleum-based lubes, like baby oil, mineral oil, or Vaseline, can eat microscopic holes in a condom, openings large enough for viruses to pass through. Very, very bad idea. Use lubes specifically formulated for sex.

You need a lube that will remain slippery for quite a while. I find that K-Y Jelly gets thick and sticky too quickly, but K-Y now makes two lubes specifically for lovemaking: a traditional type called UltraGel and one that gets warm on contact with air. I use Astroglide, but you might want to try a few different kinds and see which works best for you. Oh, and spit doesn't work, so don't bother.

There are also lubricants specifically designed for anal play, with numbing agents that make the first few times more comfortable. If this sounds like a good idea, surf adult Web sites or get a catalog from one of the larger companies, like Adam & Eve, Good Vibrations, or Xandria.

For anal sex, keep using more. If you find that the product you've tried doesn't stay slippery, use more, and more, and more. Except for the mess, there's no such thing as too much lubricant.

Partners need a greater level of trust to play with actual anal intercourse. Agree that if she says *stop* at any time, you will. No questions asked, no begging or coercion in any form. Ladies, unless you feel you can trust him to stop everything immediately if you say *stop*, then *don't play*.

A word about alcoholic beverages. A glass of wine or beer, or a cocktail, might make this easier for both of you, but too much alcohol will erode your good sense and eliminate her ability to consent. Without her true consent, you don't know how she'll feel the next day.

How to Give It for Him

If you and your partner are interested in anal sex, begin slowly. Touch her anal area gently during foreplay and gauge her reaction.

She might shy away at first, but keep trying, especially when you're both really excited. And sober. If you think she's truly against the idea, however, forget it. You don't want her to be nervous every time you make love. And please don't try to wear her down by continually pressing the issue. If you do, she'll be just as likely to reject the idea of sex with you altogether.

Once she's enjoying the feel of your finger near her anus, you can progress to insertion of a finger or a toy. Use lots of lube first, then slowly press one finger just a bit and see how she reacts. A slender anal dildo or vibrator is a great way to take this next step. Anal dildos and vibrators have a wide flange at the base to keep them from slipping into the colon. Please, please don't use anything without one. The vagina is a closed system, so that nothing can slip too far in to be retrieved. Not so with the anus. I know I'm repeating myself, but it's important to remember that the rectum is the opening to the entire digestive system; something pushed in too far can get lost. Not only is it embarrassing to show up at the emergency room needing help in removing something, but it can be extremely dangerous as well. Take care!

For cleanliness, you can cover the dildo with a condom, easily removed later for vaginal play. Again use lots of lube and slide the toy in slowly, allowing her body time to get used to the feeling. Be ready to withdraw it at any time. Once the toy is fully inserted, withdraw it slowly and press it in again to simulate intercourse. If she's enjoying it, this play should arouse her still more. You might want to add to her arousal by describing the scene and telling her how hot it's making you too.

Once you've played with a finger or toy, you're ready for actual penile penetration. By now, you're both very excited and eager to play. You've got a condom on and you've used lots of water-based lube, so you next want to think about a good position. Spoon-style, where she lies curled up on her side with you behind, works well. It also means you can reach around and play with her breasts and clit. Play with her erogenous areas a lot before you begin to try penetration. By arousing her fully, you'll both find penetration easier.

You can also try standing, with her bent over a chair or leaning on the edge of the bed. That position makes it easier for you to part her cheeks and aim at the correct location. Once you're both used to it, letting your lady straddle you as you lie on your back can work well, and it gives her control of depth and speed.

If you miss—and it happens often—and end up in her vagina, it's okay to try again. If your condom has touched her anal area, however, remove it and put another one on. Have a large supply handy the first few times. It's easy to end up in the wrong opening.

If she finds it painful, let her know that it's okay for her to ask you to stop. This isn't an endurance contest. If you allow her to play martyr and do something she really dislikes, she won't want to play again—not the result you want at all. Encourage her to be honest and, for you, go slowly until she adjusts to the feelings.

How to Get It for Her

A thirty-seven-year-old woman wrote:

For the last four years I have been engaging in anal intercourse with the man I love and it has led to some of the best orgasms ever for both of us.

At first we talked about it and I found it arousing. He had done it years ago with another woman and found it most enjoyable, but had not felt comfortable broaching the subject with anyone since. After he described in detail what he would like to do, and ascertained it was okay with me, he began touching my anus and penetrating it with his finger(s). After we did that a few times, he asked whether the next time we made love I would be willing to try anal penetration. I said yes and he assured me he would never hurt me and he would not be upset if I asked to stop without completing the act.

We engaged in lots of foreplay and I was quite aroused. He used lots of lubricant and it was wonderful. It did not hurt in the least, felt pleasant, and most importantly, I never felt emotionally closer to him. He says it gives him the best orgasms of his life because of the tightness, and I find it most pleasurable. I would hate to see anyone who desires this denied the opportunity to try it, but obviously it depends on both parties.

A thirty-one-year-old woman wrote:

I love my husband very much and had never done anything anal before I met him. He is rather large in the basement area so it took some time for me to fully relax with him inside me, even vaginally. However, after three beautiful children we found that there was little grip down there anymore so we started to experiment with anal sex, with his finger at first, then a small vibrator.

It was at this time we started to do a little bit of swinging but had promised each other no penetration would take place. I spent an evening with a very handsome dark-skinned man who took a long time performing oral sex on me then used all his fingers, which I love. I don't remember how it happened but he ended up taking me anally. I was in total heaven, but after the guy climaxed I felt ashamed that my husband wasn't the first to take me that way.

I wondered whether to tell him about my experience but I decided not to. I did, however, ask my husband to do it to me the next night. I didn't have to pretend it was my first time as he was much larger than the first man and boy did I feel it go in! I asked him to slow down as it was painful, but I don't think I ever felt him climax so hard in my life. Holy cow, the noises he made!

We now have anal sex maybe three times a week and if he's gentle I don't feel bruised inside like I used to do, although sometimes if he's feeling horny he gets a bit carried away and I feel like I have been punched in the stomach when he's finished.

My advice? Go for it and discover true sexual heaven . . . and keep your man at home where he belongs—with you!

How to Give and Get It

A twenty-eight-year-old woman wrote:

My spouse and I have tried anal sex several times now and we enjoy it more each time. I have found being on my side or on top is best. Females are into this activity more than guys give us credit for. My husband was hesitant at first about discussing it with me but one evening we were watching a tape and the guy took the woman in the rear. Well, it wasn't difficult to see that it excited my husband so I asked him. It nearly blew me away when he told me that he had always been interested but scared. Now, doesn't that beat all!

A few years later I had a male friend who wondered whether to talk to his wife about anal sex.

When he asked my opinion I encouraged him do it, immediately. I told him that you really have nothing unless you can be honest with your spouse. "What if she's always wanted to try too, but hasn't had the nerve to ask?" I asked him, remembering my husband. He told me later that he asked and they did it, and liked it.

A thirty-one-year-old man wrote:

My wife and I have been married for about nine years now, and I have always been more open and adventurous in trying new things sexually than she is. I like trying new things, but I'm hesitant about introducing her to anything adventurous because of her sexual shyness.

I had read articles about anal sex and decided that I would like to try it, seeing as how our sex life needed a little spicing. The first few times I would just gently rub her anus, and then I tried sticking just a fingertip in. She would push my hand away but she didn't say anything negative about my actions.

One evening we spent quite a bit of time playing and I knew she was really excited. I began running all four fingers back and forth across her vagina, moving my index finger closer to her anus each time. I did this for several minutes, getting my fingers lubricated sufficiently with her natural juices. Then I took the plunge. I stuck my index finger in her ass, still keeping my other three fingers in her vagina.

When I did it, not only did she not push me away, she actually let out a little groan. I was very turned on by this because she had never made a sound during sex before. I took care not to get the anal finger anywhere near her vagina since I'd read about the bacteria problem. I kept up my thrusting into both her openings until I felt her stomach muscles begin to tighten, as they usually do when she is reaching an orgasm, and felt her asshole begin to clench around my finger.

After close to nine years of marriage I think that was the best sex we had had. I am still working up to asking her to let me penetrate her anally. I am sure if she would just give it a try she would enjoy it as much as she did my finger that first time.

A thirty-year-old man wrote:

Just a word of advice for men who want to entice their ladies to have anal sex. Learn from my mistake.

My wife and I had done it on two previous occasions without any lubrication and from then on she was strongly against doing it ever again until this past weekend. Knowing what I know now, I don't blame her at all.

Anyway, for several months I casually mentioned it now and again and always get the same response from her. I love my wife and want it all to be good for her so I certainly wouldn't do anything she wouldn't enjoy. I'm not above continuing to ask, though. Finally this past Friday I sent her a sexually explicit photograph of a couple engaging in the act. I told her I was ready if she was and she agreed.

I woke my wife the following morning with a

long massage followed by bringing her to a pleasant orgasm. She prefers a back and neck massage to get her going more than any other method. After she was fully satisfied I began to prepare her anus and my penis for the event.

I massaged K-Y gently around and into her tight back door and slid one, then two, then three fingers into her while she lay on her stomach. I knelt behind her and—as gently as I could—pushed the head of my penis in. She let out a little whimper saying it hurt, and I stopped immediately. I told her that, if it was okay with her, I would hold still and wait to see whether it would feel better when her body relaxed. For me, the feeling was incredible, and it took a great deal of concentration to keep from exploding right then and there. Slowly I felt her entire body relax so I asked her if it was all right if I pushed a little deeper. She agreed and it was more wonderful than I had imagined. I know I didn't last very long because within a very few minutes the sensations overwhelmed me and I came. She told me that once the initial pain ended she actually enjoyed it, for herself and for me.

The next day I sent her flowers. I've vowed to myself that I'll wait until she suggests it for the next time. I think she will.

A forty-two-year-old woman wrote:
My lover and I had been talking about trying anal sex for a while, mostly joking and teasing each other. I must admit this was a new thing for both of us . . . we were "virgins," so to speak.

After reading a lot about it on the Web, I

decided to "call his bluff" the next time he teased me about it. He never pressed me, or forced me to do this; it was something I wanted to give him, a part of myself that no man has ever had. In my opinion, if you're in a relationship where there is love, trust, and respect, it can be one of the most incredibly erotic sexual experiences in your life.

We took a whole afternoon alone together, used *lots* of foreplay and K-Y Jelly, and took it *very* slowly. He was so sweet and patient and eventually we found that the "spoon" position works best for us. I was amazed at how intense the sensation was and so surprised when I had a fantastic orgasm just from anal penetration.

I feel closer to him now than I ever have. It's such an intimate and trusting act with someone you love. This act that most consider "nasty and forbidden" can be wonderful with someone you love and, most importantly, trust.

A thirty-nine-year-old woman wrote:
I have some of my best orgasms during anal sex. Perfect? Well, a few have been pretty damn good.

Until a few months ago I had always considered anal sex a taboo and would never have dreamed of trying it. My husband has always commented on what a beautiful butt he thinks I have, and every now and then a finger or his penis would stray to the "forbidden zone." Finally after discussing our feelings about trying it and reading a book about creative sex, we took the plunge and I'm happy to report that I absolutely love it.

I was terrified that I would be in incredible pain, but such was not the case. Although I had a wonderful experience, I would hesitate to recommend trying anal sex to anyone who doesn't have a longtime partner. There should be complete trust and respect between the two of you, or it could go terribly wrong.

Here's a bit of advice. Buy a very good lube. We used one called ID Glide. Use more than you think you need, and once you feel you have too much, use more! Take it slowly and arouse your partner to the boiling point. Tentatively try several positions until you find one that is mutually comfortable and has you both relaxed.

Buy some latex gloves, too, and make sure your fingernails are neatly trimmed and smooth. You'll probably want to try inserting one finger at a time at first, rather than going directly for entry with a penis, dildo, or anal plug. A small jelly butt plug is great. Having sex with the butt plug inserted is sheer heaven for both partners.

Most important for any guy who wants to try it, respect your partner's wishes. If she wants to stop, then *stop*! You can always try again another time. I won't say it's for everyone, but I will say that now I'm thrilled that I tried it.

A *fifty-three-year-old man* wrote:
I've been married to my wife and best friend for almost thirty years. I have always been curious about anal sex, but any attempts were unsuccessful due to my wife's inability to relax her anal muscles. And I didn't understand that it takes stimulation to

prepare an anus for sex. Finally I found what I consider to be the key to anal entry.

My wife loves it when I lick her pussy, and I started gently touching her anus while licking her. That eventually progressed to finger insertion, which she actually found to be pleasurable. Then I inserted my index finger into her pussy and my middle finger into her ass and in a few minutes of licking and fingering she had an incredible orgasm. The thing I noticed was that as she came and her pussy spasmed, her anal muscles actually relaxed. I ordered a few anal toys in different sizes and also ordered a new lubricant called Probe.

After a few sessions with the toys and the comfort gained with the new lube we tried again. A massage and pussy licking coupled with double-fingering her with the new lube actually had her suggesting that I "try it again, gently." To our mutual surprise the head of my cock painlessly popped into her virgin ass. After a few seconds of her trying to understand that I was actually inside of her with no discomfort she pushed back and my whole cock slid up her ass.

I was so aroused by the feel and the picture of looking down and seeing my cock buried balls-deep in her rear that I thought I would pass out. Feeling her apprehension about my starting to fuck her that way, I told her how wonderfully different it felt and just slowly moved my cock in and out. In my highly aroused state it only took a few seconds before I came so hard I almost fell from my kneeling position.

Since that time we have anal sex at least twice a month. She says it's a totally different feeling from vaginal sex and so we have each at different times.

I have even talked her into stimulating my anus
from time to time. I found I love it and I recommend that you try it too. A dildo or vibrator up my
ass and touching my prostate gives me an erection
like a twenty-year-old!

How to Give It for Her

This last letter brings up another issue. Ladies, don't overlook the
delicious things you can achieve with anal sex for him. You don't
need a penis to penetrate. Fingers and toys work wonderfully well
for stimulating his anus. Most of the same rules as those above apply.
Of course there's no danger of cross-contamination, so condoms
obviously aren't needed.

A few words about fingers, however. Ladies, if you're going to
insert your finger in his anus, take care with your nails. Make certain
there are no sharp corners or snags. Actually, you might want to
cover your finger with a well-lubricated condom to assure a smooth
surface, especially if you have long nails.

As for him, use lots of lube. For his anus you can use Vaseline or
baby oil, as long as none of it gets near your vagina.

A word about the prostate. It's a dome-shaped organ about a
finger's length into the anus, on the belly side. If you reach in far
enough, you can't miss it. A light rub can send a guy into orbit.

A sixty-eight-year-old man wrote:
Perfect is hard to define. When my lover massages
my prostate with either her finger or a butt plug
and gives me oral at the same time, I have multiple
orgasms. It's a sort of ripple effect that happens no
other way. The repeated intense peaks and release
literally make me cry out. Yeah, maybe *perfect* is
the right word.

Anal Sex

A thirty-four-year-old man wrote:

My wife and I have enjoyed anal sex for quite a while now, but recently she changed the entire game. She ordered a strap-on dildo and surprised me one night by asking me to let her penetrate me.

The dildo was very large and I was a little afraid she would hurt me, but after an extended session of pushing up to four of her fingers into me, I let her mount me.

I won't kid you, it did hurt a little at first even with her going slowly, but it was worth the initial discomfort. My wife had done this with a previous lover and she knew how to hit my prostate. I came with a climax I will never forget. Now I am adjusted to the nine-inch monster and take pride in the fact that I can take it up to its big latex balls. I love every minute of it. I highly suggest it to other anally oriented couples.

A thirty-five-year-old woman wrote:

I have been married to my childhood sweetheart for fifteen years. We have to two teenage boys and live a happy suburban life. Behind closed doors, however, we are not the quiet family others see. We enjoy all kinds of sex. He has penetrated me anally, with fingers, tongue, and penis, and we enjoy it immensely.

However, he has always been reluctant about being penetrated, and I was pretty sure he'd enjoy it if he would just relax and let me. Well, eventually we started a journey toward his anal penetration. I've always enjoyed erotic stories and I used them to bring the subject up to him. Beginning with stories that I knew would arouse him, I began to tell a few while I performed oral sex on him. He came particularly powerfully that night, so I knew I was on the right track.

Next I began to insert one finger into him during blow jobs, and eventually he got to the point that he allowed me to use a small strap-on. Each phase of the journey added to our trust and enjoyment. His orgasms seemed to escalate as we progressed. My orgasms seemed more intense because of the trust he placed in me. We talked about each phase before we proceeded to the next.

Of course all the foreplay and lubrication standards for anal sex with a woman are required for men as well. As a woman I truly believe the act of penetration was empowering. I felt like I was given a gift, and I treat it as such every time he lets me strap on and thrust in. We have found a new strap-on that stimulates me much better, and I look forward to our first simultaneous orgasm.

A twenty-five-year-old man wrote:

I think anal sex is a fantastic thing, and a complete surrendering of one's self to someone you trust. However, there's one angle on it that I haven't seen much talk about: women performing it on their man.

My ex and I had a very sexual relationship—it was the one thing we did very well—and after a while every time we were going at it doggy-style, she'd reach back and rub my anus with her fingers, which always brought me to climax in short order. We talked about it and I said how I'd engaged in anal masturbation in my single days so she took it to heart. One night during sex she rubbed her fingers over her soaked pussy and inserted a finger into my anus as I thrust into her from behind. It was intense.

Gradually we progressed until one day we ordered a strap-on off the Internet for her. The first time she put it on I went crazy seeing her with this translucent seven-inch latex cock strapped to her. We got into the mood pretty fast and after some foreplay and lubing my ass, I straddled her as she lay on the bed, grabbed the strap-on, and inserted it. It was intense riding her "cock." She took me doggy-style then and after an hour or so of various positions I reversed the situation and took her anally. The whole night was fantastic.

So lesson of the day is that enjoyment of anal sex is something men and women share. Trust me, it's worth it. I'd recommend that a woman try it with a strap-on, especially one with a smaller vibe or dildo attached to the harness for her pleasure so she gets the penetration sensations as well.

An eighty-three-year-old man wrote:

I am an eighty-three-year-old man who wants to try everything for as long as he can. In this case, several years ago, I suggested that my wife first digitally explore my backside by explaining to her how doctors examine men rectally to determine prostate size. A middle finger inserted deeply into the anus and pressed downward as the man bends over a tabletop will find a walnut-sized object. That is the prostate. Stroking this ball-like organ can actually lead to ejaculation, which is quite pleasurable for both participants, although embarrassing if it occurs between doctor and patient. For couples it can be an extension of the adolescent nurse and doctor game, and, in my case, has led to further explorations with dildos.

How to Get It for Him

A thirty-six-year-old man wrote:

To any man who wants to suggest that his wife anally penetrate him, here's my suggestion:

The best way to approach her with it is to ask her about her own fantasies. Emphasize that you want to hear the really "dirty" or "nasty" ones that she's never shared with you before. If she shares them, it's a huge bonus for you.

Whether or not she does, she is almost guaranteed to turn the tables eventually and ask you about your fantasies. If you think she would be too put off by your desire (which I doubt she would if you are close), challenge her ego first by declining to tell her, because you don't think she could handle it. She will almost surely take offense, convince herself she won't be bothered by whatever you say, and demand to hear. Then tell her you are curious about anal stimulation. Gauge her responses. Be as explicit as you want within her tolerance level. You don't have to dump on her now that you fantasize about being gang-raped by a coven of strap-on dominatrixes. Tell her you aren't sure how far you will want to go, but you would like for her to try using a finger on you sometime, if she would be comfortable with it. If she accommodates you, show enthusiasm, and she will probably get into going as far with it as you would like.

A forty-one-year-old man wrote:

I had a really difficult time discussing my desire to be penetrated in the rear with my wife. I've always encouraged her to talk to me about her desires but I just couldn't tell her about this . . . until a few weeks ago.

We were watching a few XXX movies together and one happened to have a scene with a guy getting done anally by women. I gathered my courage and took the opportunity to comment that it would be exciting, then expressed interest in other scenes where toys were used on the men. I was totally surprised at how little it took for her to become eager to try one of our vibrators on me. I never came so hard.

It was exciting for both of us and we now incorporate anal sex into our lives regularly. There is nothing like an orgasm with a vibrator against your prostate. And I think most women secretly want to do a man like that and experience a sort of role reversal. Good luck.

A thirty-seven-year-old man wrote:

My wife isn't interested in anal sex, but that doesn't stop me from playing—by myself. Here's how it began.

I bought a vibrator for my wife a few years ago. You know the type—a little five-inch hard plastic bullet. Unfortunately, she promptly put it in the back of her nightstand and it was never used in our bed. This summer, while she was on a business trip, I decided to take it out, put in a fresh battery, slide a condom on, lube it up, and slip it in my back door while I masturbated.

You can't imagine my excitement when I turned it on. I exploded! Since then I have bought a jelly anal vibrator and I'm hooked. I like the feel of the little probe but when the vibrations start I can't control myself. If you guys like a little pressure on your prostate during sex—this is the same only *much* better.

Chapter 12

THE POWER OF POWER

THIS CHAPTER INVOLVES ACTIVITIES THAT NEED
a few words of warning. To begin, I need to define the term *consenting adult,* since only a consenting adult may play. And the definition may seem pretty straightforward, but it's not as obvious as you
might think.

In our society the age of consent is defined by law—eighteen or
twenty-one in most states. Well, that's not good enough here. An
adult is not merely someone who's reached some important birthday, it's someone who is mature enough to decide what's a good idea
and what's not. A twenty-five-year-old might not be old enough to
consent if he or she doesn't have a clear understanding that the word
no is an acceptable answer to any request. No amount of begging
and/or subtle coercion should be part of such a decision, and an
adult must be old enough, mentally, to understand that.

To consent, a partner must know that not consenting is an
option and an important one. Consent involves the conscious decision that *This activity is one I want to try. I might not enjoy it, but
I'm willing to give it a go.* No alcohol, no drugs, no coercion of any
kind can be part of such a decision. No "If you do it I'll love you

more." No "If you loved me you'd do it." No pouting, no yelling, no force of any kind should be part of your decision to play a new game.

In addition to being a consenting adult, if you are to play power or bondage games, or indulge in activities that involve pain, then a tremendous amount of trust must exist between the partners. *No* means *no* and that's the end of everything, no matter what, and you must trust your partner to stop. Period. Afterward, you two can discuss whatever problems you encountered and, perhaps, try again another time or adjust the game. This puts a burden on you as well. If something gets uncomfortable and a little voice says, *I would really like to stop,* you must, and I do mean *must,* say so. Don't suffer in silence. If you do, your partner can't trust that he or she isn't doing something mentally or physically painful. If you agree to say *stop* at any time, then your partner can proceed until a protest is made, confident that whatever activity is going on, it's okay with you.

Now that we have those basics out of the way, let's talk about power. Why should anyone want to dominate a partner? There is a very good and exciting reason.

If you're the dominant partner and the one in charge for the evening, then you can do anything you want, secure in the knowledge that your partner will say *stop* if anything gets uncomfortable. And I do mean *anything.* You can ask for or demand anything from an erotic massage to lengthy oral sex, from watching your partner masturbate to anal sex. You can spank, slap, berate, humiliate, anything that excites as long as all the proper measures are in place. Think what freedom!

If you're the submissive partner, the one who only follows orders, then you can relax and not think about a thing. You don't have to worry about whether you're making the right moves, in the right order, at the right time. You're being told what to do. If your partner wants to do something a little off center, as long as you're okay with it you don't have to consider society's rules. You're not in charge here. Worried about whether you know the mystical secrets of oral sex? It's not your job to know. It's your boss's job to tell you. You can even ask, "This way, master?" Delicious, isn't it!

One last thing. You might like to yell *stop* during some activity, like playing pirate and captive or guard and prisoner. How is your partner to know whether it's a genuine request or part of the game? That's where the concept of a *safe word* comes in. A safe word is one that's agreed on by both players—an unusual word that will stick out and say, "Stop now!" You can use *chrysanthemum* or *marshmallow*, or the one that those who play a bit more formally use: *red*. You can go farther and use *red* for "Stop now" and *yellow* for "Stop for a moment so we can adjust something," if (say) your foot is cramping or the rope around your wrist is too tight.

Armed with these strictures, playing power games and using bondage and pain can be fabulously erotic side dishes on the path to the perfect orgasm.

How to Get It

A fifty-one-year-old woman wrote:

> One evening many years ago, my husband and I made a bet on a football game. A last-minute fumble made him the winner. For his prize, he said he wanted me to be his sex slave for half an hour later that evening. I laughed, assuming it was a joke. It wasn't.
>
> We talked for quite a while after that and got some rules worked out. I wasn't sure I wanted to play this way but I trusted him to stop at any time so I agreed. Actually, the whole idea was quite exciting for me despite my reservations.
>
> Later in the evening, we went upstairs and my husband set a timer for half an hour. "Until this

goes off, you're mine," he said with a theatrical leer. "Now strip. Very slowly."

I'm not too happy with my body. I'm at least thirty pounds overweight and I seldom let my husband see me naked all over. I was shocked that he wanted to look at me. Well, I stripped, awkwardly I will admit, but he didn't seem to care. His eyes never left my body and he looked as though he was aroused by the view. I never thought he'd enjoy seeing me without clothes.

When I was naked, he gestured me over and told me to unzip his pants. Well, out sprang his fully erect cock. The "show" I'd just put on must have really gotten to him. He grabbed me by the hips and pulled me down on his legs. There we were, him sitting on the edge of the bed with me straddling him, my large breasts in his face, his hard cock lodged deep inside of me.

Well, it was heaven for me. All I had to do was raise my body, then lower it when and how he told me to, while he sucked my nipples. Orgasm? You bet. One of the best ones I've ever had.

We play like that often now and from time to time I'm in charge, although he's the masterful one most of the time. It's just fabulous.

A forty-three-year-old man wrote:
When we first married my wife was very shy. She'd never been with another guy and was really hesitant about doing anything other than the missionary position. I found it a bit frustrating, but I loved her and so I was willing to wait until she was more amenable.

After about a year we had a long discussion

about our sex lives and she admitted that she was afraid to try new things, sure she'd do something wrong and embarrass herself. I said there was nothing that I wouldn't like but still she demurred. I thought about it and, several weeks later, suggested that we play a little game. She was to be my employee and I was her boss. She was on the verge of being fired and had to do anything I said to keep her job. At first she thought it was silly, but eventually she decided to play along.

I sat at the kitchen table and we pretended it was the desk in my office. I began by telling her what an inferior employee she was and that she'd have to do something really special to keep her job. She asked what she could do so I showed her. I pulled off my jeans and briefs and sat back down. I pointed at my crotch.

My wife had never performed oral sex on me before so I made it as easy as possible. I'd taken a shower so I knew I was pretty odorless. I told her to get down on her knees and service my cock. She looked like a deer in the headlights. "I'll tell you exactly what to do." And I did.

First I had her lick me like a Popsicle, then kiss the tip. She readily did what I asked, seemingly enjoying what she was doing. I thought I could go a bit farther so I asked her to hold it while she put the tip in her mouth. It felt so good that I pushed her away and came with her still holding my cock with her hand.

Well, that was just the beginning. I've instructed her (we both love that term) in exactly how I like my cocksuckers (we like that term too) to behave, and she's become an expert on exactly what I like. Now that we've come this far I can't wait until we branch out into other things.

How to Give It

A thirty-one-year-old woman wrote:

I love to keep my lovers on the edge of climax but not let them get there until I'm ready. Let me explain a little bit. I'm the boss in all my relationships. I have several lovers who thoroughly enjoy my ministrations, and each knows he's not the only slave I have. It's all just sexy fun and games. Every evening, before we play, we reinforce the idea of safe words and such.

We begin with dinner out and sometimes a movie or walk. The longer my guy has to think about what's coming up, the more comes up, if you get my drift. Usually, by the time we get to my place, he's really hot and ready for his "torture."

First I make him strip, then he puts on a pouch, one that is at least a size too small. That keeps his mind on his cock, as if it might be elsewhere. I've taught each man how I like to be loved and I only date guys who are good learners. I can stretch out on the bed for a massage, or sit spread-legged on a chair for lots of good licking. From time to time I'll squeeze his crotch or scratch his testicles with my fingernails.

Most of my guys like me to use a butt plug on them. I make them bend over a chair and spread 'em so I can insert a well-lubed dildo, then I put the strap of the pouch over the flange so it stays in place.

I keep this up for exactly as long as they want and I always know when they are reaching their limit. At that point, sometimes we fuck, sometimes I watch him get himself off. It's always great for him. I make sure of that. And of course it's great for me.

A thirty-six-year-old woman writes:
This might seem really silly to you, but my husband and I play hypnotist and patient. It began as a role-playing thing when he helped our older son with a report on the history of mesmerism. We came into the bedroom after putting the kids down and he waggled his fingers at me and muttered "You are getting sleepy" a few times. In play, I collapsed on the bed and pretended to be under his spell.

He gave me a few silly instructions, then told me that I was getting really horny. I really was, just from the game. We fucked like wild people and, when we were recovering, he gave me a posthypnotic suggestion: When I heard the word *hydrangea* I would be back under his control. Now we play about once a month. It's really fabulous.

Bondage

Bondage is one of the supreme demonstrations of power. Having your partner at your mercy can be an extreme sexual turn-on for both parties. In the previous section I spoke about the allure of either being able to demand any kind of sexual pleasure or just following orders. Being bound or having your partner tied up intensifies these feelings.

While trying bondage, it's more important than ever that you turn up your personal radar and tune in to your partner's reactions. If her eyes glaze over with passion, you can carry on to the next step. If, however, you sense a pulling away from the game, then stop. Reinforce the need to use the safe word and assure your partner that you trust her to say *stop* and that you will respect her wishes, no hard feelings.

How to Get It

In many of the preceding sections I've talked about communication and how to ask for what you want. Bondage is one of the most difficult topics you can bring up, but once you do, the sky's the limit.

To get around the "he or she" problem, let's assume she will be bound and he will be the one in power. If you're on the opposite sides, merely reverse the genders as you read.

How can I ask to be bound? That will ruin what I'm looking for—the spontaneous surrender of power. Well, you can't ask for spontaneity. If you ask for what you want today, however, you might get the spontaneousness in the future. You have to start somewhere.

How do you bring it up? Try this: During lovemaking, lift your arms above your head and, if only in your mind, pretend you're restrained in whatever way you fantasize about. Or when you're both really aroused say, "Maybe I can't move . . . can't keep you from doing whatever you want to me."

How to Give It

During lovemaking, hold her wrists lightly, not to frighten, just to give her the feeling that you're restraining her. To do it in a light-hearted way, try saying, with an overdone leer, "How would you like to become my sex slave?" Keep it light and nonthreatening. Maybe, while playing cards or Scrabble, you can suggest that the loser will owe the winner an hour of bondage.

Play bondage by creating a story in which she is bound. Stretch her arms over her head and say, "I've got you tied to the bed, so don't move." Or "I gave you something in your drink before and it renders you helpless, unable to move." That way you can gauge her reactions without getting into actual ropes or chains.

Rent a video that presents the subject with a light touch. You might want to prewatch it to be sure it doesn't get into anything heavier than you have in mind. Then watch it together. If your partner shows any sign of being interested, pursue the matter. "Would you like to do something like that? I think I might be interested."

Erotic stories can take the place of a video. Print one from the Internet or write one yourself. It doesn't have to be good, just hot. Of course, you can use any of the letters in this book as well.

Once it appears that your partner might be open to the idea, then you can begin the fun. There are lots of ways to play with bondage without actually really restraining anyone. For starters, you can use thread to tie your partner. She can break it at any time, but you both can experiment to see how you both like it. At a moment of passion, he can also say, "You have a twenty-pound weight on each wrist and so you can't move either arm."

When you're ready to restrain your partner, you don't have to get fancy with bondage equipment bought from a store or Web site. Use things you have around the house: panty hose, neckties, the sash from a robe. Keep it soft and sexy. Slide it over your partner's body first to demonstrate its softness and strength. Take advantage of anything that happens.

A forty-one-year-old woman wrote:

It all began one evening when I tried to remove a wad of hair from the bathtub drain after my shower. Somehow my hand got caught and I yelled to my husband for help. I knew that if I just relaxed, my hand would come loose, but it was a bit of a scary moment.

Anyway, he came into the bathroom and there I was, naked as a jaybird, with my hand stuck unable to move. Well, he teased that he could do anything he liked with me trapped that way. I found that pretty exciting, despite my predicament. I laughed and told him to just get my hand out. He started to help but the area was still wet from my shower so he first removed his shirt and jeans.

So there he was, bent over me so I could feel his hardness against my back. He was quite obviously really hot. So I took the plunge. I wiggled my behind against him and said, "What if I never got loose? I guess we'd never have sex again."

I think he was startled but he stopped trying to grab my stuck wrist and thought for a moment. Then he said, "We could have sex this way and you couldn't do anything about it, could you?"

I think the word *could* was his way of asking. "I guess I couldn't," I said, and that was enough for both of us. He reached around and grabbed my breasts, hanging over the edge of the tub, and pinched my nipples. It was the hottest moment of our marriage. He fucked me in that position.

As I collapsed on the bathroom floor after one of the best orgasms of my life, he noticed that my hand was free from the drain. "Oh," I said, "it came out quite a while ago, but I didn't want you to stop."

From then on, control in one form or another played a large part in our relationship. At least once a month he ties my hands to the bed or to my thighs with lengths of soft nylon clothesline we bought together at the hardware store.

I noticed lots of types of chains there too. I think I'd like that and I might suggest it to him the next time we're looking for something new.

A thirty-one-year-old man wrote:

My new girlfriend had played bondage games with her ex and she told me about it. She said she had the best sex ever while tied up. I had often looked at pictures of bound women on the Net but I would never have dreamed that a girl-friend of mine would be interested. I thought it would make a woman feel like some sort of sex object but my girlfriend seemed to really want to be tied up.

I thought about it for quite a while, not really sure I would like it in real life. One evening we were walking through the mall and wandered into the pet shop to look at the puppies. Right beside the cages was a display of dog and cat leashes, collars, and such. She looked at me in that way she has and picked up two cat collars and two narrow leashes, took them to the counter, and paid for them. Totally dopey, I said, "We don't have a cat."

"You have me," she said with that tone in her voice. Needless to say I couldn't wait to get her home. When we got to our apartment she fastened one of the collars around her left wrist then asked me to buckle the one around her right. Well, that was all the invitation I needed. I accepted that she really wanted it.

We quickly undressed and went into the bedroom. I fastened the two leashes to the head of the bed then clipped them to the collars around her wrists. That way she was not bound tightly but her arms were prevented from moving too far. Then I straddled her and demanded that she suck my already very hard cock, something I know she loves to do. She gave me the best blow job I've ever had.

The next weekend we went back to the pet shop and bought several of those choke-chain collars for dogs and got a few small padlocks at the hardware store nearby. Now we play often. Thank heaven she was brave enough to bring it up.

A fifty-two-year-old woman wrote:

I tie my husband up often and he loves it. Ladies, you can always tell by the hardness of his cock, and my husband's gets like steel.

We had been doing it for several years and it had gotten pretty routine. Then I was looking at bondage sites on the Net and realized that there are so many more ways to tie someone up than just four points (you know, wrists and ankles tied to the corners of the bed).

I got some new, very soft, nylon rope and cut it into five-foot lengths. For lots of evenings after that

I tried different ways to tie him up. Here are a few of the ones we particularly enjoy.

I have him sit in a chair and I tie his calves to the front legs and his wrists to the back ones. Then I tie his elbows behind him. One time I tied his wrists together in his lap, then put on one of his favorite porno movies. I told him that if he touched his cock I wouldn't have sex with him. I loved to watch his cock twitch with his hands right there but not able to relieve his itch.

One evening I tied him stretched facedown over our coffee table, arms and legs tied to the legs of the table. Then I teased him with a butt plug. God, he came like gangbusters. Then he performed oral sex on me for about an hour. It was wonderful.

Moral? Don't just do the ordinary. Be creative.

A fifty-six-year-old man wrote:
This might sound medieval but my wife and I have a playroom with a set of stocks I made to work like ones I'd seen in a movie. I'm pretty handy and I have a wood shop in my basement but it took several weeks and a few mistakes. Eventually I'd made the kind that hold both your head and wrists. I also made a bench for her to sit on at just the right height. I want her immobile, not uncomfortable.

After a few sessions I cut most of the seat from the bench so I now can play with her pussy while she's being punished for being a "bad girl." I'll never forget her delighted surprise when she realized what I'd done. I think she must have come a dozen times that night.

It's amazing how many times a week she's "bad." I'm smiling now just thinking about it.

Spanking

Pain as pleasure might seem really bizarre, but many people find that a swat at the moment of climax increases the pleasure. Others find that, when their bottom is sensitized with a few spanks, it makes the genitals extra sensitive as well.

How to Get It

A thirty-five-year-old woman wrote:

I've been married for eighteen years to the same wonderful man. About two years ago I was looking on the Internet (you gotta love the Internet) and found several sites that seemed to say that people enjoyed spanking their spouses and the people receiving the spanking actually enjoyed it. I found the idea really turned me on, but I was ashamed of my feelings and didn't mention it to my husband for several months.

Eventually I got up the nerve and finally told him what I'd been thinking. I said it kind of joking but he surprised me by saying that he was curious too. One evening, as I was about to climax, he slapped my bottom a few times. I came really hard but that wasn't exactly what I wanted. I found myself more and more interested in a bare-bottom, over-the-lap spanking and I told him so. He was dubious, but a few evenings later he did it. Sadly, his spanks were so light that I barely felt them. I think he was more afraid of hurting me than anything else. I assured him I would let him know if I was being hurt and that I wanted him to really do it so I could feel it.

It took a while for him to get into it but I think my excitement spurred him on. He now realizes that I really do enjoy to be spanked hard and that if he gives me this kind of pleasure he is in for a treat as well.

A few nights ago he wanted oral sex. I was okay with it but I wanted a spanking. I would suck for a few seconds then stop and finally he asked what I wanted and I told him a spanking. So he did. In return he got the most excellent blow job he had ever had. I am not one to swallow and had only done it once before but he got me so excited with the spanking that I just could not stop sucking so I swallowed every drop. Since that night he has spanked me several more times and I believe he has enjoyed it as well.

A fifty-one-year-old man wrote:

Goddamn it! I just found out what all the fuss about spanking is. I have been wanting my wife to spank me to see whether I liked it and today she finally did it. Did I come! Just from the spanking alone, rubbing my cock against her thighs as she pounded my ass. I am so happy. My wife is now a triple threat—she can fuck me, give me a hand job, or spank me to orgasm. I am so fucking happy.

A *thirty-three-year-old man* wrote:

I love it when my wife spanks my ass. Hard. And while she does it, she holds my cock between her thighs. It's wonderful. Recently she turned me over her knees and stuffed an anal probe up my behind before she spanked me. God, I thought I'd died and gone to orgasmic heaven. Perfect? Maybe the best I've ever had.

A *fifty-year-old man* wrote:

I don't know what came over me recently but I guess it began with my reading stories about spanking starting at a young age. The idea always titillated me. With the advent of the Net, I found spanking sites and used the pictures and stories when I masturbated.

My wife is a very passive person but despite that I occasionally swatted her bottom as she was coming. It seemed to me that she came extra hard and I wondered whether she might enjoy a real spanking, but I never worked up the courage to suggest it. Until a few weeks ago.

She was going to be away from home for several days on a business trip. We both travel a lot so we plan special time before a trip, calling it a going-away present. For some evil reason, I asked her if she intended to touch herself while she was gone. She actually blushed, then said she wouldn't but her tone of voice suggested she wasn't taking the question very seriously. I said that I thought she needed some incentive to be a good girl while she was gone. I got up from the bed, and came back with a hairbrush from the chest of drawers. I told her to roll over on her stomach, and I placed two pillows beneath her hips. The fact that she was cooperating gave me the courage to go on. I then took the belt from my housecoat and tied her hands above her head and straddled her thighs.

Suddenly her entire demeanor changed. She softly told me to stop. I asked her if she really meant it and she thought about it for a minute then whispered, "No."

I'd read enough stories about this kind of thing that I knew about safe words, so I said, "If you want me to stop just say *uncle*."

She said it and I knew she'd remember.

Well, she never used the word. As a matter of fact her sharp intakes of breath and comments, like "Ooh that stings," and "Oh, please don't hurt me," spurred me on. From time to time I reminded her that the safe word was *uncle*, but she just said, "No, please stop." I grinned, looked at the pinky red hue of her ass cheeks, felt the heat of her skin, and grinned.

Finally, after about six hard slaps, I put the brush aside and placed my fingers against the hottest, wettest vagina I'd ever felt. I couldn't believe it so I got really serious and said, "You really want this, don't you?" When she nodded slightly, I continued to stroke her and said, "You want me to spank you more, don't you? You want me to really give it to you, right?" Her soft "yes" nearly had me coming in my pants.

I gave her six more, but then I couldn't wait any longer so I untied her hands, rolled her over, and thrust into her. We both came, screaming.

I feel so lucky. Happy are those couples who

can grow over the years to realize such satisfac-
tions. We haven't talked about it since she's
been gone but she comes home from her trip
tonight. I wonder what she'll say when I ask her
if she was good? We might need to discuss the
safe word again.

OBSTACLES

Chapter 13

BODY IMAGE AND EXPECTATIONS

WE'VE SEEN WHAT GOES INTO A PERFECT ORGASM but, sadly, there are lots of pitfalls along the way—traps that we, as questors, need to be aware of and need to know how to avoid. The sad part of the body image craze, which seems to now be affecting men as well as women, is that your feelings about yourself can seriously undermine your efforts to improve your sex life. If you don't feel good about yourself, how can you feel sexy?

Body Image

I probably receive more letters from people who are worried about their bodies than any other topic.

- "I'm a small-breasted woman and I'm considering breast augmentation surgery. As a teen my chest was referred to as two raisins on a bread board and I'm not any bigger now."

- "I'm a large-breasted woman and I'm considering breast reduction surgery."

- "I'm worried that my penis is too small and I'll never be able to satisfy a woman. How can I make it larger?"

- "I had a woman tell me that my cock is too big and that it hurts her when we make love."

- "I'm seventy pounds overweight. I want to wear sexy lingerie but I know what I look like."

- "I'm too thin and I hate my body. I'm all angles and no curves."

And on, and on, and on.

I would like to rant on about the silliness of worrying about size, but I thought my writers could say it better than I ever could. I could include hundreds of letters, but I've chosen only a few. Please take them to heart, no matter where you are on the size spectrum.

Ladies, let's begin with the baggage you carry along with your view of the way your body looks.

A twenty-three-year-old woman wrote:

As woman in her twenties I have been battling to win the weight loss war for at least a decade. I'll let you know if I ever win! It saddens me to see what people put themselves through to lose a few pounds. I am currently working on a project for a health and wellness class at my college. I have read about body wraps, yo-yo diets, "magic solutions," and whatever else the weight loss industry can entice us with. I think if I never lose the weight, oh well. I'm not gonna spend the rest of my life fretting about it anymore!

Body Image and Expectations

A forty-one-year-old woman wrote:

I have a teenage daughter who's obsessed with her weight. I talked to her doctor and now my daughter's getting counseling. I always thought that it was her peers and TV commercials that gave her the idea that she had to weigh eighty pounds, but as time passes I realize that I'm a lot to blame.

I've always been overweight and as I listen to myself at the dinner table, food and calories seem to be all I ever talk about. Sadly, I've passed this on to her.

For the women out there, take care how to think about your own body lest you pass your obsessions on to your children.

A fifty-one-year-old man wrote:

I married when I was in my early thirties and before that I dated short women, fat women, thin women, and tall women. They were all beautiful, and I mean that in the physical sense.

My wife of almost twenty years has lost and gained gobs of weight and has now settled somewhere in the middle. All I care about is that she is happy. Of course I am not physically attracted to every woman, but a few—or even a lot of—pounds is not going to weigh heavily on my mind (no pun intended!). This whole hang-up that women have with their bodies just makes me ill.

The most adorable, loving woman I ever dated was chubby and beautiful. Her cheeks were rosy with life, her smile was beautiful, and she had a heart of gold. I would rather spend my entire life with somebody like that at my side than with a "perfect ten" who constantly asks me, "Is my butt getting too big?" So I married her.

I don't care how big your butt is. Just believe you're beautiful and, like my wife, you will be. And stay away from those horrible diet pills. Is it really worth poisoning yourself just to look thinner? Sex appeal comes completely from within.

A forty-seven-year-old woman wrote:

I'm really saddened by all the hype about how women should look. So many women are so unhappy. To hell with it all. I look like an average woman, a bit overweight, saggy from the years and three pregnancies, and I don't care. I love me and my husband does too. What more is there?

A fifty-three-year-old man wrote:

I have a few things to say on the topic of body image. I grew up in an era with somewhat different notions about what women should look like. As preadolescents, my friends and I lusted after Marilyn Monroe, with her curvaceous, lush glory. We would have died laughing had we only known that some day the pop culture image of the ideal female would be top-heavy while looking like a teenage boy from the waist down. I still find it rather bizarre.

Nature designed women to be wide hipped for a reason. Until relatively recently, slim-hipped women had an unfortunate tendency to die in childbirth. Moreover, men have traditionally found female curvy hips and posterior to be a strong attraction, and in many cultures they still are. I'm sad that that's not true in ours.

Many men, like me, look for curves and soft bodies. Sexy women should look like those wonderful nudes the Old Masters painted with flesh on their bones, soft breasts, and hips. How many women condemn themselves to torture and dieting trying to look like a supermodel, and if they are successful (and at what cost?) they only diminish their sex appeal?

I've been happily married for quite a number of years to a woman who weighs more than twice what I do. Prior to meeting her I dated both thin and fat women, and although I found some skinny women attractive, it just wasn't the same.

A forty-nine-year-old man wrote:

Over the last few years I have developed a theory that you may find interesting.

I go to a health club twice a week and use a stair-stepper or elliptical exerciser and sometimes out of boredom I look at the women. These are all strangers and I realized that there are some that I look twice at. I began to consider those women and tried to find a common denominator that attracted me. Now, keep in mind that these are women whom I have never seen before and have no intention of ever meeting, plus I see them from a distance and do not hear their voices.

Over several weeks, I decided that the common factors that made me look twice at them were not their size or weight, how skimpy their exercise outfits were, the size of their breasts, their cleavage, or their ass.

There are two common denominators. One is

their smile. Just look in *People* magazine or *Playboy* and you'll notice that every celebrity and/or model has a nice smile. They seem happy to know you're looking at them, and happy within themselves.

The other thing that attracts me is a woman's posture and how she carries herself. All the women who I look at more than once seem to be self-assured and pleased with the way they look, however that is. I think there's a lesson here.

A *twenty-four-year-old woman* wrote:

I am a college-educated woman who is just plain big. I am six feet tall and weigh just over three hundred pounds. I wear a size twenty or twenty-two. I have spent the last five years fighting my weight, fighting my body image and fighting the fact that I live in Southern California where the blond bombshell is all too common.

Last year I decided to quit being a victim to my own fat. Once I accepted myself and found my self-confidence and self-worth, the amount of attention I started getting was amazing. I know I'm beautiful, and men do too. I carry myself differently and my outlook is different. And my sex life was fabulous.

Now I have found the most incredible man. When we met he told me that he usually isn't attracted to what he called BBWs—he explained that it meant big beautiful women—but he said that there is something about me that is different—and I know what it is. I love myself and it makes all the difference in the world.

Body Image and Expectations

If it's not their body as a whole, ladies worry about the size of their breasts. The ones with large breasts want to be smaller.

A thirty-seven-year-old woman wrote:

I have big breasts and I hate them. Somehow, in the dating scene, I've become a chest and not much more. I get to talking to a guy and he's really busy trying not to stare at my tits. Ugh! The guys I want to be with are the serious ones, with real brains and opinions. Somehow, those men are often intimidated by the size of my breasts. I'm seriously thinking of having breast reduction surgery. I've even made an appointment with my doctor to begin gathering information.

Ladies, if you've got a normal-size chest, or even a small one, be happy. You know guys are interested in you as a person, not a mother figure.

A forty-three-year-old woman wrote:

I had breast reduction surgery last year and I've never been happier. My back pains are almost gone and I fit into normal-size clothes. Men? I'm dating now and have been since my divorce ten years ago. I've noticed that I do get fewer first looks, but I seem to get just as many dates. The operation has been a godsend.

A twenty-eight-year-old man wrote:

I don't know what all the fuss is about. I love a woman with small breasts. I do like large, prominent nipples, though. I love a woman who can go braless so I can see her nipples through her clothing. Wow, it gets me hard just thinking about it.

On the other hand, there are women who have small breasts and long to have larger ones.

A thirty-six-year-old woman wrote:
> I had breast augmentation surgery done last year and it's the best thing I have ever done. I can actually call it life changing. I'm very weary of comments about how natural is better—well, no kidding, but some women do not "recover" from breast-feeding the way others do. After breast-feeding the last of my four children a few years ago I was left with very droopy, misshapen, odd-size breasts. To think I would have to spend the rest of my life looking at them like that was depressing.
>
> My husband never said anything negative and always told me my boobs were just fine but that didn't help. I have always taken great care in my appearance with lots of exercise and healthy living and here I was with these weird things hanging off my body. They didn't even feel like they were a part of me.
>
> Now seven months after the surgery I'm a firm, full C cup and my body feels and looks very real and natural. My husband can't keep his hands off me so our sex life has greatly improved. Yes, I would have loved to have stayed with my natural breasts had they not changed. It would have saved me a lot of money and discomfort but that was not my reality and thankfully I live in a time when a miracle such as this is possible.

A thirty-nine-year-old man wrote:

> My wife is almost completely flat chested and I
> love her, and I love her body. I really don't care
> what size she is. She's talked about having surgery
> to get a bigger chest but I've always dissuaded her.
> I love, like, and admire her just the way she is.

Amazing, isn't it? Large-breasted women want to be small and vice versa. Ladies, try your best to be content as you are. The grass is always greener in the other person's pasture. Cliché? Sure. But the reason a saying becomes a cliché is that it's true.

Here's an exercise for you. Sit in the mall and look at the women around you. Are they all perfect tens or even sixes? Probably not. Now think about your friends and acquaintances. Are all the good-looking ones happy? Are all the average ones miserable? I don't think so.

Next, take a good look at yourself in the mirror. Find your best features and concentrate on them. Let those be the last things you look at when you leave the bathroom. Say to yourself, *I've got great eyes,* or *beautiful hair,* or *really pretty hands.* Play to your strength and try to minimize your weaknesses, both in reality and, more importantly, in your mind. Have you and your partner ever made love in front of a mirror? Mirrors are a great lovemaking accessory, and if you have less-than-wonderful feelings about yourself, you'll see very quickly that your partner really doesn't care. He's making love with a warm, willing, wonderful woman. You!

Lastly, when you're next making love, look into your partner's eyes. What do you think he sees? Your faults? I doubt it. The fact that you're hot for him right now? You bet.

Sadly, in the image department, men are no different. Of course most of them don't worry about the size of their bellies or thighs the way women do, but an amazing number of them obsess about their penis, both its size and its look.

A twenty-one-year-old man wrote:

My penis is only four inches when erect. I checked a Web site and it says that I'm just at the bottom of the normal range, which goes up to about eight inches. I'm afraid I'll never find a woman who will want to have sex with me.

A forty-eight-year-old man wrote:

Although gigantic equipment may go a long way (no pun intended) in the male shower room or on a porno film, in my opinion the myth of bigger being better is just a lot of sizzle and no steak! Although it's always an interesting topic of discussion I'm convinced it doesn't matter.

I'm of average size, seven inches or so erect and decent circumference, and my wife of twenty-six years and I have great sex. It's all in the foreplay, and I'm proud to say she reaches orgasm about 90 percent of the time. We kiss sensuously, fondle each other, lick each other, even periodically use a six-inch battery-powered vibrator to stimulate her while I tend to other areas with my hands and mouth.

Quite frankly most times, if I've done my job correctly (truly a labor of love), by the time I penetrate she's so close to coming that I could be two and a half inches long and only as big around as my pinkie and she'd still explode.

A thirty-six-year-old man wrote:

I'm a healthy mature male who has always had a voracious sexual appetite that's mostly unfulfilled. I have a much bigger-than-average penis, and guys, please believe me when I say that it is not always a desirable asset. Rather, it can be uncomfortable for both your partner and yourself when it comes to insertion, especially if your woman is not really wet.

I have had more complaints about my size than I have had compliments. I suppose I should say that although I measure a full nine inches when totally erect, it is my girth that seems to cause the major discomfort. I have had more than my share of sexual experiences, mostly after I was divorced, and almost inevitably the woman first looks delighted, then wary, and eventually like a deer in the headlights. "Will that really fit?" Some don't say it but most think it, and while I prepare to enter them I can see the wheels turning. I get a woman really aroused and use lots of lube, of course, but many times it's a bit of a struggle.

So if you have average, or near-average, equipment, be grateful, and remember that bigger is not always better.

A fifty-seven-year-old man wrote:

I have one of those below-average-size penises. I have had many lovers over the years, most of whom were more than satisfied with what I could do. Three lovers who were into anal sex felt it was just the right size for a comfortable back-door ride.

Maybe to compensate for my "package" over the years I have made a point of learning what pleases a woman during sex. Some men never seem to figure it out, and some blame the size of their equipment. Hogwash.

Of course I have known a few women who said they enjoyed a much thicker instrument pleasuring their vagina, and we usually found creative ways to satisfy that urge. Cucumbers, really thick cucumbers, work great. Big butt plugs work as well in a vagina as they do on an anus. Bananas are also effective, and nothing is quite as tasty as a banana eaten right out of a vagina. I have used a variety of thick dildos, including strap-ons.

My penis isn't the thickest or longest cock on the block, but my lovers and I have put it to pleasurable and happy use over the years.

A twenty-eight-year-old man wrote:

I am a male and I have a small penis. If the average is six inches then I have about four, maybe five at the best of moments. I have managed to have some fantastic sex in my lifetime because the biggest sex organ is the brain. If the lady is really up for the big bang then the size of the penis is truly not terribly important. Of course I'm not going to star in any porno movie but who wants to. I want a warm, willing woman whom I can make so hot that when I enter her she thinks I'm Prince Charming.

Let me put in a word here for those men who feel they need bigger equipment. Forget it! I've received dozens of letters from men who've tried herbs, exercises, and various torture devices to increase the size of their penises, to no avail. One man said that, after three months of using some device or other, he gained a quarter of an inch. It had been painful, and a month after he stopped using the equipment his penis was back to its original size. Men, save your money, time, and energy and spend them on learning how to satisfy a woman. Men who can use their hands, mouths, and toys to give a woman pleasure will never want for dates or sexual evenings.

Men also seem to be hung up on the idea of adult circumcision. Should they? Shouldn't they? Again, let's let real people speak for themselves.

A forty-six-year-old man wrote:
>Few women realize how sensitive the foreskin is. When rolled down, the inner side is several square inches of very exciting tissue. It responds to stretching and pulling rather than the gliding feeling of the head. Women always go for the head, I guess because it's a bit like their clitoris. Both can produce an orgasm either separately or combined; in combination it's doubly wonderful. Circumcised men can really only have half the pleasure.

A twenty-one-year-old man wrote:
>I am uncircumcised. I have been giving some thought to having the procedure done for some time now. I have, however, upon further investigation, concluded that there is no foreseeable advantage in circumcision for me.
>
>Personally, the aesthetic reasons are the main drive for me to have the procedure done, but that alone is not enough to convince me to go through with it. I have recently come to the realization that it really doesn't matter what your penis looks like, just that it is clean and healthy. And the women I've been with don't seem to care at all.
>
>People have been saying that size doesn't matter.

Well, then why should a foreskin? (Perhaps not the most brilliant of analogies, but it suits.) I guess what I'm trying to say is that any man should be proud to have a penis, in any shape or form, and furthermore, be proud to be a man.

Remember, gentlemen, keep your head held high and walk tall.

A sixty-nine-year-old man wrote:
I feel very badly for the men who are circumcised. I can't imagine enjoying sex as much without the foreskin sliding back and forth. Also, having a fore- skin means the penis has many different looks. This makes for some enjoyable viewing for both sexes. I am soon to be divorced and I'm sure glad that I am getting back into dating with my foreskin intact.

A fifty-two-year-old man wrote:
I was not circumcised when I was born, and all during my youth I was embarrassed about my sta- tus. When I was twenty-five years old, my wife said, "If it bothers you that much, get circum- cised," and I did. It was the absolute best thing a could have done for myself. I feel much more self-confident because I look like all the other guys and during sex I like the feel of my newly revealed parts.

I tend to believe that circumcision is not med- ically necessary, but it sure helped me when I got circumcised. I don't feel like I've lost any sensitiv- ity, and I sure do like the way it looks. It turned out to be a very good choice for me.

A forty-five-year-old man wrote:

Until the age of thirty-nine, I was uncircumcised. I loved having sex and I made love with a woman with my foreskin retracted as much as I could. That feeling aroused me very much.

Then I met my current wife and for religious reasons she asked me to be circumcised. I had the operation, which was no problem at all. My only problem was that, during the healing process, it was hard to control my erections due to the new sensation (and the stitches).

After a few weeks, my penis was fully healed and we gave it a try. Wow, what a feeling, I could feel a lot more and it seemed that my penis hardly fit in my skin. After a while the excitement of this has diminished somewhat.

Masturbation is different too. Before, I rubbed the head of my penis while rolling my foreskin up and down, and that's not possible anymore. Now I masturbate holding the shaft of my penis, and the tightness of my skin echoes through to the head of my penis and is very exiting.

My wife definitely prefers the new model and says that she now can feel the head of my penis better than before. And what's more, we both love the looks of my new penis.

Expectations

Oh, those sex scenes. We read about the perfect orgasm. We read how it's simultaneous or the best there ever was, and that's despite the fact that she's a virgin or it's their first time together. And, of course, there's no mess. I hate all those scenes because they give such a monumental false impression.

Once in a blue moon, an evening with a new lover culminates in the most fabulous orgasm ever, but that's rare. Very rare. Perfect orgasms take practice. Of course, the practice is wonderful and, with any luck, the climaxes get better and better. But fireworks every time? Earth-moving orgasms in the carriage on the way to the prince's castle? I think not.

Set your sights on the perfect orgasm but be willing to work at it—to take the time, risk the communication, open yourself up. Otherwise you'll constantly be disappointed.

Premature Ejaculation

It's happened to most men at one time or another, and for the most part it's not an ongoing problem. You've probably been there, done that. You are so aroused that, when you've barely gotten started, bingo. You're done. Embarrassing, but you can get past it. Why does it happen occasionally? An exciting woman, very long foreplay, no orgasm for quite a while—all those factors can end up with a man coming more quickly than he or she wants.

For some, however, it happens more frequently. They ejaculate quickly most of the time. It might be purely physical or it might be training. Training? Sure. When you were younger and masturbated you were always on the lookout for interruptions, so you trained your body to react quickly. Now you're ready in a flash and gone in a flash.

For those of you who come too quickly for full sexual satisfaction, I have a few suggestions:

- Masturbate to ejaculation before lovemaking. You will probably find that a second erection lasts longer and you'll climax more slowly.

- There are commercially available products that slow down arousal, and they work. How? Most are numbing agents, like lydocaine or benzocaine. You rub the cream on the penis and it mutes all sensations, usually slowing down orgasm.

- If you don't wear a condom, wear one. If you already wear one, wear two. That will have relatively the same effect as the numbing agent and, in addition, it will act like a cock ring to slow down return blood flow from the penis.

- Cock rings also work. They are attached around the penis and testicles before arousal and, like the snug-fitting condom, they keep blood from flowing out of the penis.

- You can also try doing Kegel exercises. I'm told that these exercises, usually recommended for a woman to tighten her vaginal muscles, can help men develop the muscles they need to maintain an erection. Kegels are simple to do. I know I'm repeating myself, but guys need to know this too. While urinating, use your muscles to stop the stream. Those are the muscles you're going to be working on. Do that several times until you can clench and release these muscles at will. Now do so, both quickly and slowly. Do it for several weeks, increasing the duration of the contraction and the speed with which you tighten and release. After several weeks you should notice a difference.

- Retrain your body. Try to get to the edge and pull back. It's not easy, but try to feel when you're approaching the point of no return. Try to gauge the moment just before that and stop anything that arouses. Keep doing this and you'll train your body to take its time.

There are other things you can do to improve your lovemaking without actually addressing the problem directly. Make sure your partner is satisfied:

- Play for a long time before penetration so she's also ready to climax almost immediately.
- Bring her to climax before insertion with your hands, mouth, or toys.
- Bring her to climax after you've come. Don't decide that, because you've ejaculated, love-making's over. There are myriad ways to please a woman that don't require an erect penis, so learn some.

Practice, practice, practice.

A thirty-one-year-old man wrote:
When I was a teenager I used to come at the most embarrassing times with a partner, and without much stimulation. I thought the problem would

wear off as the years passed, but it didn't and I still come much too quickly for my taste. I've learned to be a good lover despite this, however. I have had a lot of sexual relationships over the years and I always make sure the woman is satisfied, either before intercourse or after. Most women never realize that I've come too quickly. Well, maybe they realize, but I don't think they really care as long as I make it clear that I'm satisfied and make sure they are as well.

Women and Menopause

Menopause causes various symptoms that can affect a woman's sex life. Hormonal changes at midlife can alter our response to sexual arousal.

Some find that, with the passing of the problems of birth control and the sudden appearance of an empty house in which they can yell as loudly as they want during sex and play in every room without fear of embarrassment, their libido shifts into overdrive. Others find that the lessening of hormones means their libido goes through the floor.

The simplest solution used to be hormone replacement therapy. I took hormones for fifteen years, and the HRT regimen completely reversed the effects of menopause, including hot flashes, vaginal dryness, and so on. Then a study came out that seemed to show that HRT was harmful. Like many other women, I stopped. Cold turkey.

So now I too have to deal with the side effects of lower estrogen levels. Many women switched to phytoestrogen—plant-based estrogen products—but for me that wasn't to be. I get migraines, and all those over-the-counter products are headaches-on-the-hoof for me. I had to find other solutions. Unfortunately I had to learn to live with the hot flashes, which did decrease in intensity and frequency over the months that followed. However, I will say that, two years later, my thermostat is still a bit out of whack. Ed's become used to me throwing the covers off in the middle of the night.

Other symptoms, like vaginal dryness, can be dealt with. Been there, done that one. Don't hesitate to use a commercially available lubricant and try to get past the *I'm not wet so I'm not aroused* bugaboo. It's not the lack of arousal that causes a decrease in wetness; it's just physical. I asked Ed many months ago to use lube during intercourse, and I've been training my knee-jerk mind not to associate my level of wetness with arousal. Get past it, ladies. It's just physical. I've discussed lubes in several sections of this book; flip back to the sections on condoms or anal sex if you need more information.

The drop in libido is another issue. Sadly, for the moment, Viagra is recommended only for men, and there are no similar products for women. There are, of course, as many infomercials advertising cures for "mature women" and their lower interest in sex as there are miracle cures for baldness. Save your pennies (and your dollars). Most are phytoestrogen, hype, and clever marketing and packaging. Since sexual arousal is as much mental as physical, you might find they work for a while, but because the FDA doesn't regulate any herbal product you've no idea about the long-term side effects. Discuss it all with your gynecologist. There are new developments every day, and with baby boomers approaching menopause, more and more will be done. It's a zillion-dollar market that the drug companies will quickly exploit.

Again, if you are experiencing any sexual dysfunction, lessening of the libido, inability to climax, and such, schedule an appointment with your doctor. And if you find it terribly embarrassing to discuss sexual problems with your doctor, try your best to get past that. He or she has heard it all before and will probably have suggestions to help. Don't give up!

Part of the problem is that the expectation of failure creates a self-fulling prophecy. You expect to have a drop in sexuality, so it happens. So much of libido is between the ears, not between the legs. Try new things, or reenergize the old ones. I think the key word here is *try*. You've got so much to lose.

How to Get It

A seventy-one-year-old man wrote:

As a man of seventy-one whose wife is sixty-nine, and with neither of us taking hormones or any other product, here is how we have mutually gratifying sex. Shortly after age fifty, with onset of menopause, my wonderful wife lost 80 to 90 percent of her libido. We talked about it and I told her how important sex is to me. We used lube and, in the beginning, I think she did things just to please me. Gradually, over maybe a year or so, she began to realize that she wasn't just giving me pleasure, she was getting pleasure herself.

We started using a vibrator, too. Now she applies a vibrator to her sensitive areas with her hips elevated on a firm pillow while I enter her from the scissors position with our bodies at a ninety-degree angle to each other. This angle of entry enables my penis to contact her g-spot. She usually has two or more orgasms before I have a powerful one.

Our lovemaking isn't as frequent as it used to be. We probably average doing this about every other week and I masturbate two or three times per week but it's worked out well. We still feel satisfied and as close as we ever were.

Medications

Several medications affect either the libido or the ability. Antidepressants and blood pressure medications are prime among them.

Antidepressants

Sadly, antidepressants tend to depress the sex drive while they are doing their job with your stress and anxiety. They make you content and less interested, or they make the body willing but unable. Please see your doctor. It might not have to be that way. Sex is important to both physical and mental health, and your doctor will be the first to admit that. If you, male or female, are taking an antidepressant, and it's decreasing your feelings of sexuality, see your doctor and ask whether you can switch to a different medication. Different chemicals have different results for different people; there just might be one that has less of a libido-depressing effect.

A thirty-two-year-old woman wrote:
> I have been married for a little over ten years now. Seven years ago my doctor discovered a chemical imbalance after I had a heart-wrenching miscarriage. He prescribed an antidepressant called Wellbutrin, which did nothing for my depression and totally eliminated my sex drive.
>
> I had always had a very high sex drive and

previously I had never, ever had a problem in that area. It took only a short time for my libido to crash. I couldn't have cared less about sex, and when my husband and I made love, orgasm just didn't happen. After about two months of this I told my doctor. His reaction? "That's not good at all." I loved him for that.

Anyway, he switched me to Paxil. It was heaven sent. Within the first week, I was feeling so much better and my husband noticed the difference too. Sex was fun again.

I can happily say that I never had any sexual side effects with Paxil, and I am still taking it. I have sex with my hubby several times a week and it's never been any better.

So to all those women or men on antidepressants, here's what I recommend. First, make sure you're on the right drug. Then, instead of trying to achieve that orgasm quickly, get into the mood slowly, read sexy stories, watch sexy movies, look at sexy magazines. Love yourself, literally. Touch yourself, enjoy your body; you know what feels good. If you think more sexually, every day, trust me, you will reach that high-interest point again.

Note: This woman's experience doesn't mean these particular medications will work or not work for anyone else. I know of folks for whom Paxil was a downer and Wellbutrin became the drug of choice. Please, consult your doctor and keep trying.

Blood Pressure Medications

Blood pressure medications don't work on the mental side of sexuality, but the physical might let you down. Erections are based on blood flow to and from the penis. If the blood pressure is lowered, a man might not be able to get or maintain an erection. I'm told that some have sexual side effects for a woman too. Again, please seek medical help. Changing the medication or the dosage might just do the trick.

On Viagra and Other Products

Before we talk about Viagra, let me burst the bubble for all of you who think you can and should get herbal products that work as well. Take care. First, most of the stuff you can buy as a result of some e-mail spam you received is powdered junk. Since so much for our sexuality is mental, you might find that you take the stuff and it works. So would a sugar pill.

That's the least that can happen. There are several widely advertised products that folks take without any regard to long-term effects. Who knows whether, after taking it for a year, your penis falls off? Okay, maybe nothing that drastic will happen, but you have no idea what you're putting into your body, guys.

Oh, and buying prescription medicine on the Web can result in you paying good money for counterfeit pills. You don't know what you're buying. I know those miracle drugs are expensive, but it's worth it to get the real thing. Believe me. I know from personal experience.

Miracle of miracles, Viagra works. In this next section I'm going to talk about Viagra, but there are two other products that have similar effects, Levitra and Cialis. Men, talk to your doctor about which might be right for you. According to the advertisements, Levitra works more quickly and can be taken on an empty stomach. Cialis is said to last much longer than the four hours of the others.

All three have several very tricky drug interactions. Ed is taking a medication for prostate problems and was accidentally prescribed Cialis, which reacts very badly with it. Fortunately the problem was realized before he took any of the medication. Read all the literature that comes with any product and check with both your doctor and pharmacist.

Viagra and its friends are a miracle, a recent medical advancement that can make a gigantic difference to the man who doesn't get rock hard anymore, or who never has. Let me tell a story from my personal experience.

Ed and I have been together since 1984. As of this writing I'm sixty-two and he's sixty-six. We've had great sex and learned how to please each other in ways we had only dreamed about when we met. We've explored toys, role playing, storytelling, and many other things I talked about in this book. Then Ed turned sixty-six. For quite a while, my sexual pleasure hasn't been what it had been previously. My orgasms had become more and more irregular, happening maybe every fifth time we made love. Oh, I got tremendous pleasure out of lovemaking, pleasure from Ed's pleasure and from my own, but climaxes? Not as often. The change occurred so slowly that I rejected the idea that there was a problem.

What was the reason for my lessening of orgasmic pleasure? Ed has never been a rock-hard kind of guy, and it never bothered either of us. As the years had passed, however, his erections became more problematic. Often he would lose his erection while we were making love, only to regain it five or ten minutes later, after more playing. Our lovemaking would finally end with his climax, but by then my pleasure had peaked and I was on the downside of enjoyment. My ability to time my own pleasure waned. I found myself frustrated, either because I'd come and wanted to just cuddle, or because he lost his hardness, the thing I needed at that moment to climax. In addition, most of the time I crave hard, fast intercourse to bring me to climax and, at the critical moment, Ed's penis wasn't hard enough for what I wanted. We managed, of course, but I wasn't getting nearly the pleasure I had in the past.

Although I encourage couples to talk about problems like this, I said nothing. Ed has never had performance anxiety, but I didn't want to create a problem. I fell into the trap I see with so many other relationships. Ladies, if Joan Elizabeth Lloyd, author of a dozen books on sex and relationships, couldn't discuss a problem, I certainly can't fault you for the same thing!

I had thought about Viagra, of course. Viagra. For people who can't get it up. That's what sexual dysfunction and Bob Dole's television commercials meant to both of us, and that wasn't Ed's problem. He always got an erection; it just wasn't necessarily a complete one. And he climaxed almost all the time. Eventually.

Finally, several months ago, when Ed was about to have his annual checkup, I gently mentioned Viagra, not knowing whether it would have any effect on my difficulty. "I don't need it," he said, totally unaware that I had the problem, and why not? I had never said a word. "Our sex life is fine with me. Sometimes my body doesn't cooperate, but it's really okay." Even then I didn't tell him that it wasn't okay with me.

Fortunately, Ed mentioned Viagra to his doctor, and she gave him a sample. He didn't tell me about it, worried that it would taint his "experiment."

One evening about a week later we made love. It was better than it had been in a long time. It wasn't drawn out as it had been when he had to stimulate himself to erection for a second time in a session. His cock got hard and stayed hard, and we "fucked like bunnies." I didn't know why, but he did. "How do you like Viagra?" he asked me as I tried to catch my breath.

"You got some?" I asked, totally nonplussed.

"Sure did. Like it?"

Hell yes. It was fabulous for both of us. He was harder with more reliability than he had been since—well, to hear him tell it, since ever. And I had the type of intercourse I needed. Viagra was a miracle.

How does it work? Frankly, I don't know, and I'm not going to research it and then bore you with scientific explanations. Your doctor can do that, or you can look it up on the Web. What it does is really quite simple. It makes the penis harder during erection. It's not an instant hard-on. Arousal is needed. It's not an aphrodisiac, creating unstoppable sexual urges. As a matter of fact, Ed says he feels no different after he's taken the little blue pill, either before or after it's begun its work. It just means that, when aroused, the penis responds more aggressively. It doesn't hasten ejaculation, but it does enable more forceful thrusting. It doesn't seem to shorten the refractory period, the time a man's body needs to rest before he can become erect again, but we're still experimenting with that—evil grin.

Taking Viagra changed things, and it was not an easy transition. It's necessitated lots of discussions and changes in our patterns. Let me explain.

First, we invented "Date Night." For obvious reasons spontaneity isn't going to happen. It takes half an hour or so for the pill to take effect, so we have to decide beforehand whether we are interested in making love that evening. Declaring Date Night means we're both interested. Of course, he could take a pill every night, but at five dollars a pop, that's really not an option, and that's not the way Viagra was designed to be used anyway.

I worried about Date Night—would it mean we'd be making decisions at six o'clock that would carry over until ten? Surprisingly, it's worked out wonderfully. Remember when you were dating in school? You and your partner knew that Saturday night was "the night." Did it spoil it for you? I doubt it. You were like animals in heat, waiting for Saturday. Maybe you went out to dinner and couldn't eat a bite. You knew what was coming (and who was going to come) later that evening. It was delicious. Well, that's what Date Night is like for us.

If you are considering Viagra, talk with your partner. Discuss the changes that it might bring to your sex life. Does she want it? Maybe she's found that things are just the way she likes it without any help. You two really need to talk. A lot.

A *fifty-one-year-old man wrote:*

> I was in a sour marriage and toward the end of it I had to masturbate to get hard enough to penetrate my wife. As soon as I was 80 percent erect there was an urgency to "put it in." I would come soon after insertion, a feeble, weak orgasm.
>
> After we divorced I compulsively masturbated for six months. I guess I was trying to convince myself I was still virile, but the fear of failure and performance anxiety kept me from even attempting to find a lady to just date, let alone have sex with. I have always had a very strong sex drive and this increased my frustration. I was in a downward spiral, getting worse each day.
>
> Well, I met a divorced lady I liked whom I felt comfortable with, and we started to date. We were both golfers so we always had something to talk about. After three dates she made it clear that she wanted to sleep with me. I resisted—I was sure I could not perform. She invited me to her house the following Saturday, telling me that her daughters would be with their father for the afternoon and we would be alone. More panic.
>
> I decided then and there to do something, so I made an appointment with my doctor—regarding anxiety. I wasn't about to tell the receptionist it was for impotence, and I wasn't impotent. I just

had problems getting really hard. It wasn't sexual dysfunction.

I insisted the appointment be soon and it was set for that afternoon. I had five hours to sit and rehearse what I was going to say to the doctor. "It works sometimes." "Well, less than sometimes." "It never happened before so it must just be my bad marriage." Et cetera. I was in a panic while I was sitting in the exam room, waiting.

The doctor walked in and asked how I was doing and I blurted out, "I would like to try Viagra."

To my complete surprise he didn't look at me any differently, he merely said, "Okay. Your heart and blood pressure have always been fine so I'll write it for fifty milligrams, and I suggest you try a smaller dose, twenty-five milligrams, until you find what works best for you." Did I worry over nothing or what?

Well, I showed up at the lady's house about noon on Saturday after already swallowing the little blue pill. The first thing my lady friend said was that she was very nervous. *You don't know the half of it,* I thought. She gave me a tour of her home and the last stop was the bedroom. We started undressing and then she lay facedown on the bed with just her panties on. Naked, I crawled over to her and pulled off her panties and then, as I knelt over her straddling her butt, blood started pumping into my penis in a way I was unfamiliar with. It just kept pulsing and pulsing. I had an erection in just a few seconds. My penis worked again! I became immediately relaxed and did not have that urgency to "put it in" right away.

I gave her a gentle massage, starting with her neck and shoulders and slowly working down to her thighs, not missing anything on the way. I gave her a pat, and said, "Roll over to the fun side." As she turned over, she saw my erection and said, "Oh . . . wow." We made love for thirty minutes and I had the strongest orgasm I have ever had. After the orgasm I stayed erect for another five minutes so we continued until we were totally exhausted. We lay next to each other for another five minutes and I still had more of an erection than I had when I masturbated to try to get one.

Later we sat in her kitchen drinking a beer and having a couple of smokes. I was naked and she was too, except for her panties. She said she needed to tidy up because her ex was bringing her daughters home in an hour so she went to the sink and started to clean the glasses. I watched her butt jiggle and thought how erotic that was. Well, I barely tickled my penis for a few seconds and had another full erection.

Seeing me that way, she said, softly, "I'm sorry we can't do it, the kids . . . I hope you understand." I got dressed and drove home with that fabulous hard-on. I still use Viagra, but there are times when an erection happens without it. I never realized how much pain this kind of sexual dysfunction had caused me until it was gone.

A fifty-four-year-old man wrote:
I've been taking blood pressure medication for several years now and it has been making it difficult to get hard enough to penetrate my wife's vagina. I used to look at nudie pictures and do anything

kinky I could think of to get hard. I even shaved my pubic hair to get aroused.

I would get semi-hard and if I concentrated I could get hard enough to get inside her, but then I would come and she'd be disappointed. She thought for some reason that she no longer turned me on. Our bodies were changing from when we were younger, but I still loved her and I told her over and over that my feelings hadn't changed.

Finally I talked to the doctor and she gave me Viagra. It works! It doesn't work anything like the jokes talk about. This is how it is for me.

I take the stuff and wait an hour or so. If Momma is in the mood, we start kissing and touching each other's body. She touches my penis and it starts to respond, just like always. But—big difference—it gets not just 70 or 80 percent hard, it gets *hard*. Then, as I slip it into her vagina, it gets even harder. With every stoke, I feel it stiffening and I am in control.

Before Viagra, when I was hard enough to penetrate her vagina, I came almost immediately because it had taken all of that concentration just to get hard. With Viagra I am hard enough to get it in and I can concentrate on holding off until she has an orgasm. We love it. The stuff works for almost four hours, so we can and have done it twice in a row. The only thing I regret is that I waited so long to talk to my doctor.

CONCLUSION

WELL, I'VE GIVEN YOU SOME OF THE INGREDIENTS
you can use to build your sexual sandwich. Tonight? Lots of kissing,
straight intercourse with a little blindfolding and a quick slap on the
behind during climax. Tomorrow? Intermammary intercourse while
she's tied to the bed with a dildo inserted to give her pleasure. The
next day? The sky's the limit.

There are several points worth reemphasizing here:

- Communication is the key to improving your sex life.
  Neither you nor your partner was born knowing, so
  ask for what you want. Use the nonverbal techniques I
  discussed earlier, particularly bookmarking and body
  language. Keep your radar receiver turned up to its
  highest level. Be aware of the tiny signals that your
  partner is giving off. And partners, don't make your
  lover guess.

- Don't be put off by what you're *supposed* to enjoy, or
  not enjoy. Keep an open mind. If two consenting adults

want to indulge in any form of sexual activity, it's none of anyone else's business. If it feels good, go for it!

- Don't slip into the tempting thought that if it was fun yesterday, it's good enough for today. Yesterday you may have had a tuna on rye. Today consider egg salad, a taco, or even a bagel with cream cheese, lox, and onions. Predictability can be the death knell of a good sexual relationship.

- Don't forget to begin the fun early in the day. Anticipation can fuel an encounter, heating both you and your partner long before you get together.

- It might be embarrassing to try something new, change something that's been okay for a while, or talk to a professional about a sexual problem. Good sex is a vital part of keeping a relationship alive for ten, twenty, or forty years. Don't let reluctance hinder your efforts.

- Always be encouraging. If you discuss sex, emphasize the positive then, if you want to, suggest something new gently. Be aware of your partner's reactions, but don't back down until you're sure an activity truly isn't his or her cup of tea. If you do discover that your lover doesn't want the activity you're hot for, however, stop bringing it up. Find something different to suggest. There's so much to try.

- Feel good about yourself and your partner, and reinforce that every day. Tell him or her how much you enjoy your lovemaking sessions, and tell yourself that you're wonderful. You are, you know.

Conclusion

There are lots of activities that can kick your sex life up a notch, and I've left some out of this book due to lack of space. But if it isn't in the book and you and your partner enjoy it, or even think you might, go for it. Now! Or later after lots of teasing and play.

Whatever you do, just be sure to make the most of every sexual moment. Like food, sex is an ever-renewable pleasure. If you make a little effort, your encounter tonight can be as wonderful and rewarding as the one you had twenty years ago, or will experience twenty years from now. Have a blast.

If you want to read more about lots of the topics in this book, click over to my Web site at http://www.joanelloyd.com and peruse the forums. And please drop me a note at joan@joanelloyd.com or by snail mail at Joan E. Lloyd, P.O. Box 221, Yorktown Heights, NY 10598, and let me know what you've tried. Of course, if any questions have occurred to you while you read, please ask and I'll try to answer them. I look forward to hearing from you.